VAGINAS

Vaginas

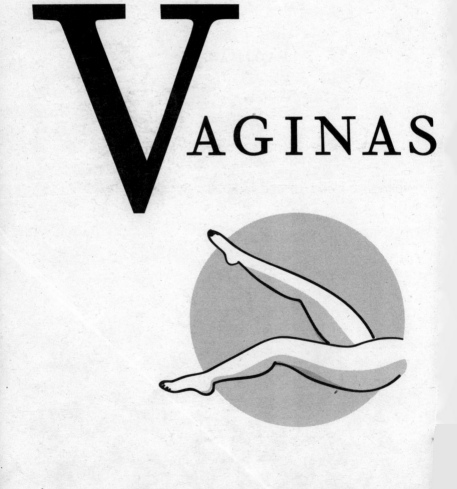

an owner's manual

BY DR. CAROL LIVOTI AND ELIZABETH TOPP

THUNDER'S MOUTH PRESS
NEW YORK

VAGINAS

AN OWNER'S MANUAL

AVALON
publishers group incorporated

PUBLISHED IN THE UNITED STATES BY
THUNDER'S MOUTH PRESS
AN IMPRINT OF AVALON PUBLISHING GROUP
245 W. 17TH ST., 11TH FLOOR
NEW YORK, NY 10011

CATALOGING-IN-PUBLICATION INFORMATION FOR THIS
BOOK HAS BEEN FILED WITH THE LIBRARY OF CONGRESS.

ISBN: 1-56858-295-1
10 9 8 7 6 5 4 3 2 1

INTERIOR DESIGN BY SARA E. STEMEN
ILLUSTRATIONS BY GEORGIA RUCKER

PRINTED IN CANADA ON RECYCLED PAPER
DISTRIBUTED BY PUBLISHERS GROUP WEST

To the only member of our family without a vagina.
We love you anyway.
Thanks, Richard.
Thanks, Dad.

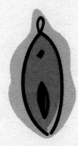

Aren't all books about vaginas?
—Y. Clete Christopher

TABLE OF CONTENTS

ACKNOWLEDGMENTS

It's possible none of this would have come together without the early support and guidance of Ron Demond Jarrett, a man whose recent career change has left publishing without one of its future stars. Thanks, Ron, for introducing us to Erin Reel, our agent who manages to be diligent, kind, and utterly fabulous, and never takes more than an hour to return a call—even on Sunday. which brings us to our editor, Kathryn Belden. Thanks for massaging our rambling dialogue into a book we can all be proud of. To Whitney Lee, our foreign rights agent, thanks for spreading the gospel worldwide. Dr. Edmund Kaplan was our first expert opinion, so thanks Eddie, for keeping us accurate. Thanks also to our second and third experts, Dr. Tom Lallas in gynecologic oncology and Dr. David Gershan in HIV. And to Katie Granger, may you proofread everything we ever write. Finally, to our best buddies: Laura, life is empty without a best friend. Kaena, thanks for telling me that everything's going to be alright.

introduction

TWO QUESTIONS

WHY DID WE WRITE THIS BOOK?

We all grow up thinking that our experience is universal. For me, that meant a Dad who cooked and walked me to school (in addition to working full-time) and a Mom who was an obstetrician/gynecologist. While this arrangement sounds familiar today, twenty-five years ago it was anomalous. When I spilled some juice on my favorite overalls at nursery school, my teacher said, "Don't worry Elizabeth. You'll take it home and your mommy will wash and iron them for you." Aghast, I replied, "*Iron?* My mommy doesn't know iron!?!"

Instead, Mom knows everything about the female anatomy. As I entered my teen years, it occurred to me how unusual our family was. In the midst of what seemed like perfectly average "how was your day" conversations over dinner, female friends of mine would sit slack-jawed as my mom recounted patients' stories, especially complicated surgeries, medical politics. Many of these friends went on to change their lifestyles, from choosing particular contraceptives to altering their exercise regimens, on the basis of my mother's candid discussions.

I've been bugging my mother to write this book since I was fourteen. Her intense dislike of computers and her inability to focus her thoughts linearly were significant roadblocks to the project. So at twenty-seven, as an aspiring writer, I thought what better than to collaborate on a project that will deliver powerful information (and, hopefully, entertainment) to women everywhere. So here, finally, are stories and information from a seasoned gynecologist, as told to her daughter.

WHY DID YOU BUY THIS BOOK?

The majority of women will never see their own vagina. It's not conveniently located for viewing, and many feel that once they've rigged up the mirror, secured some privacy, girded themselves for some unexpected surprise, well, after all that, why bother? These same women will inspect each gaping pore on their faces, every groove in their fingernails, and each errant hair; but the vagina and its environs remain unclaimed by their owner, examined by others but left alone most of the time. We'll start with the assumption that you, reader, do not know what your own vagina looks like. Even if you are among the bold few (congratulations!), the majority of your reproductive apparatus remains hidden from view.

Discomfort with one's body is not limited to seeking out your own nether regions in reflective glass. While many conventions are relaxing, the reality for women remains that nudity outside of the bedroom or bathroom is unusual and discouraged. Western women will often look East and tsktsk other cultures for carrying feminine modesty to a twisted extreme, but we needn't look that far. Opportunities for women to see other average, naked women are few and far between, even in our modern but still modest culture.

Contrast the female experience with her genitals to that of a man. His entire journey of reproductive self-exploration can be conducted by simply looking down. At an early age, boys are thrown into environments where nudity is the norm. In 1993, my private high school in New York City opened a brand new gym in which the men's locker room had a communal shower while the women were given stalls. It may not seem like a profound discrepancy, but it demonstrates how boys learn that there's a natural range of sizes, widths, colors, and hair distribution

Vaginas

among male apparati. Women are left to compare themselves to pictures, television, and movies, where, for the most part, you can forget about seeing vaginas anyway (and if you did, they'd be hairless).

Consider that for their entire walking lives, men are not encouraged but required to handle their penises several times every day. They stand, dick in hand, between strangers at urinals. Surely, they need to achieve significant levels of comfort with handling their own genitals, and from there, it's not such a long way off before they learn other fun things they can do with their penises.

The situation is surely improving, but girls are often discouraged from touching "down there." Like everything with vaginas, masturbating is not so intuitive for us ladies. And orgasms, while sometimes difficult with a partner, may just be impossible if you don't know your body well enough to get yourself off. Is it any wonder that women feel somewhat dissatisfied in their skin, and particularly, about their vaginas?

It's difficult for us to learn our bodies. There is so much mystery and culture tied up in vaginas and the rest of the equipment that enables human reproduction. While others have attempted to dissect the intricate web of social, anthropological, and emotional issues with regard to female genitalia, we have somewhat less lofty goals. This book is a manageable primer, peppered with stories from the forefront of gynecology, tempered by the perspective of a single, urban twenty-something. Here is a guide to your equipment, how to keep it running, how to tell when something is going wrong, what to do about it, and also, how to have fun with it.

* * * * *

MOTHER: "Isn't this a very short chapter?"

DAUGHTER: "It's fine for now."

MOTHER: "Are all the chapters going to be this short?"

DAUGHTER: "No. We can come back to this one."

MOTHER: "When?"

DAUGHTER: "Later."

MOTHER: "Why would we come back to it?"

DAUGHTER: "I don't know, Mom. Can we move on now?"

MOTHER: "Oh, okay. Sure."

DAUGHTER: "Just stay calm."

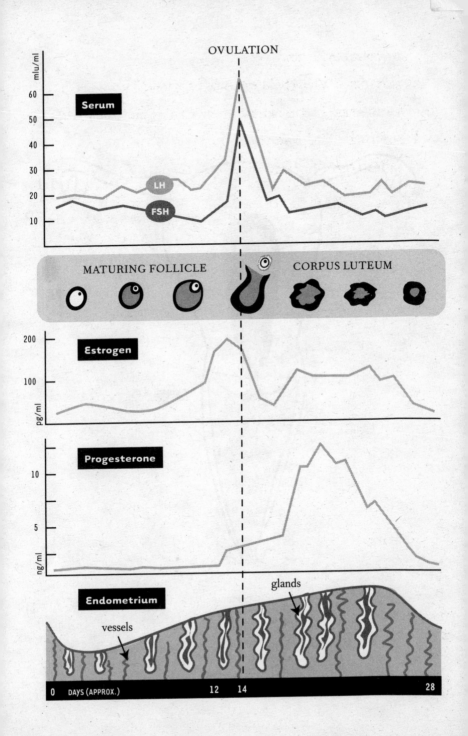

OVULATION

Serum

mIu/ml

LH

FSH

MATURING FOLLICLE   CORPUS LUTEUM

Estrogen

pg/ml

Progesterone

ng/ml

Endometrium

glands

vessels

0   DAYS (APPROX.)   12   14   28

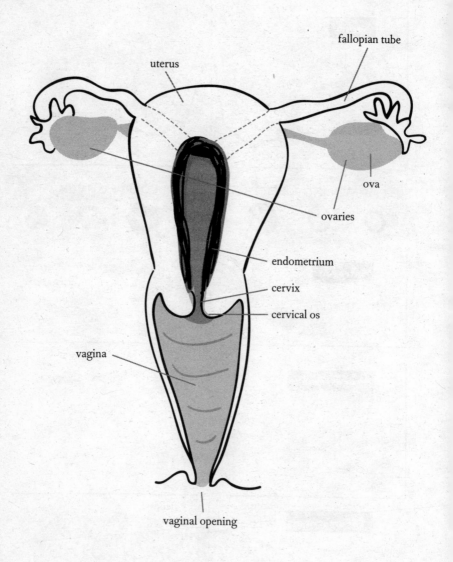

uterus

fallopian tube

ova

ovaries

endometrium

cervix

cervical os

vagina

vaginal opening

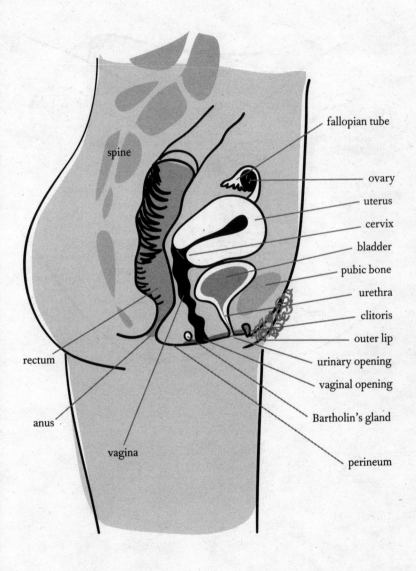

fallopian tube

ovary

uterus

cervix

bladder

pubic bone

urethra

clitoris

outer lip

urinary opening

vaginal opening

Bartholin's gland

perineum

spine

rectum

anus

vagina

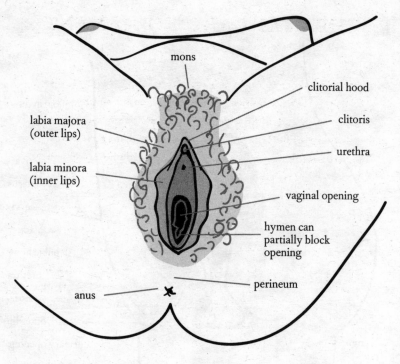

mons

clitorial hood

clitoris

urethra

labia majora
(outer lips)

labia minora
(inner lips)

vaginal opening

hymen can
partially block
opening

anus

perineum

chapter one

THE STANDARD EQUIPMENT

For most women, vagina talk is discomfitting. We rarely discuss the relative hairiness, smelliness, color, or size of our
genitalia, because there's very little to compare ourselves
to. And there just aren't enough euphemisms to describe
what seems, at best, inappropriate for the dinner table and,
at worst, gross.

I had a friend when I was about twelve who wore panty
liners every day of our very athletic summer camp. They
looked extraordinarily uncomfortable to me, and when I
asked her why she bothered with them, she blushed,
shrugged, and said, "I just don't like *it*." Well, for her and all
the other women out there who can't stand the fact that
their vaginas seem messy, that's a healthy vagina you've got
there. Stop cleaning up after it, and let it be.

You reach full gynecological maturity in your early twenties. This
means that your cervix is mature, periods are regular, ovulation happens the vast majority of the time (90 percent if not more), you're fertile, and your breasts are fully developed. You are ready physically, if
not emotionally, for motherhood.

OVARIES

The ovaries (AKA female gonads) are analogous to the male testicles.
Ovaries are squishier than balls and they're only about three by two
centimeters. They float in the abdominal cavity, attached by ligaments
to the side of the uterus and the pelvic wall. Ovaries have no surface

A patient came in reporting "ovulation pain"—the same pain she gets at the same time every month, only it was the wrong time. I kept assuring her it was almost certainly not her ovaries, but she insisted on disagreeing with me. A week later she called back with the exact same pain, and I assured her it could be any number of things but it certainly was not a week-long ovulation. Finally, she went to her local doctor who diagnosed kidney stones. Trust me, abdominal pain is usually not your ovaries.

barrier, and are therefore unprotected from their environment, just as the environment is unprotected from them (see page 201).

The female gonads consist of connective tissue (stroma) and vessels. Dotted throughout the stroma are tiny fluid filled sacs called follicles. Each follicle is made of hormone-producing cells that cradle a single egg. We are born with all the follicles we'll ever have (see page 145 for an interesting development). They remain dormant until the early stages of puberty, at which time they start to produce hormones. Each month, one lucky, proactive follicle explodes into the peritoneal cavity releasing an egg. The site of the ruptured follicle ultimately heals but leaves a small mark, so eventually the ovary looks like a soft peach pit.

The ovary is arguably the most precious organ of the reproductive tract because it contributes to our entire female shape, mood, libido, and health. Furthermore, the eggs contained within are the only way for us to pass on our genetic heritage.

TUBES

The fallopian tubes are pipes that act as conduits for eggs and sperm to meet, which they do, in a normal situation, at the outer third of the fallopian tube. So the earth moves in the tube. The tubes are very delicate structures that can easily be injured. The openings to the tube, called fimbriae, are wispy. They look very much like fronds of seaweed floating in the ocean. Fallopian tubes are about three or four inches long, and vary in diameter, getting skinny in the middle and wider at either end. They don't do much, except act as the road to reproduction.

Some researchers think that the fluid in the tubes is a nutrient for the developing embryo as it swims down to the uterus, and furthermore, that this is an integral part of the reproductive process. A lot of time and money is currently devoted to learning about the environment in the fallopian tubes, so that we can duplicate it in test tubes for in vitro fertilizations.

THE UTERUS AND CERVIX

Your uterus (without a fetus in it) is about the size of a plum. The cervix is about a three-centimeter continuation of the uterus. Together, they look like an upside-down pear.

The unoccupied uterus doesn't do much. Strictly speaking, it doesn't make any hormones that anyone cares about or knows about. And yet women invest a whole lot of emotion in it. To many, it symbolizes womanhood, femininity, or maternalism. Just as the heart really is a multichambered pump, it's also a symbol of love.

The uterus has three layers. From inside out they are the endometrium, the myometrium, and serosa also known as peritoneum. The endometrium is the lining that plumps up and then sheds every month during childbearing years. And thins and becomes inactive after menopause. It's where embryos embed. It's also what doctors scrape when they do a D&C (Dilatation & Curettage—a common diagnostic and/or therapeutic procedure where the gynecologist dilates the cervix and scrapes the inside of the uterus with a slim, flexible spoon called a curette). The myometrium is the muscle. It expands when you're pregnant, and contracts when you have cramps or contractions. It's thick and strong. The serosa is the smooth and shiny layer of tissue that covers all the organs and surfaces in the abdomen, including the uterus. Its function is to prevent everything in the peritonal cavity (the hollow space below your diaphgram) from sticking to everything.

The cervix consists of connective tissue, squamous and columnar epithelium. The cells that line the cervical canal are called columnar epithelium, which has nooks and crannies like an English muffin. It's one cell layer thick and produces mucus that helps the sperm get to the uterus. The connective tissue keeps the cervix closed and prevents it from opening at the wrong time. The squamous epithelium covers the part of the cervix that faces the vagina; it is the same lining that covers the whole body (i.e. epidermis). It stretches, it breathes, it excretes, it protects, it's waterproof—nature's Goretex. It is many cell layers thick, and at the cervical opening is the squamo columnar junction (commonly called the S-C junction), where the columnar cells meet the squamous cells. This junction plays an important roll in your gynecological health (see page 232 for more details).

THE NEIGHBORS

If one assumes that specialization of function (meaning that different organs have a specific, unique function) is a sign of advanced evolution, then the human female is the most advanced animal on the planet. We have three perineal orifices to the male human's two, all three of which perform different tasks: one for liquid waste, one for solid waste, and one for reproduction. Men use one orifice for both liquid waste and reproduction.

The Cervix as a Pregnancy Test

There are loads of old ideas about the cervix and how it behaves during pregnancy. A doctor in the fifties might have said, "The cervix looks a little blue, you're pregnant." Or if your cervix is too soft, you're pregnant. Or if you can bend the uterus onto the cervix, you're pregnant. Nobody under eighty years of age knows any of these tests. They're just not done outside of the most alternative medicine circles—go to a pharmacy, get a pregnancy test, pee on a stick, you'll know (almost) for sure.

@vaginas

That's the good news. The bad news is twofold. Our "holes," if you will, are so close together, cross-contamination can be a real problem—meaning that some of the stuff in our vaginas, for example, isn't so good for our urethra. Our orifices were designed for a quadruped, meaning that all of these perineal pathways would be better off if they were parallel to the surface of the earth, and therefore relatively immune to gravity's pull. Now, thanks to evolution, they are vertical so gravity can act aggressively upon them. In summation, the orifices we have are nice in theory, but in practice, they're not so hot.

THE URETHRA

For starters, the urethra is too short. It is only approximately one inch from the outside world to the bladder, which is a very easy climb for bacteria. It only takes an hour or two for an industrious bug to get from start to finish. A man's urethra can be eight inches long (or so they tell us).

We've all heard the phrase, "Stop making me laugh, I'll pee in my pants." This fear is shared by three-year-old girls and eighty-three-year-old ladies alike. A few muscle fibers create an angle where the urethra joins the bladder. The muscles act as a closed door when you are standing, but when those scant muscles deteriorate, it can be a challenge to hold your urine in, and you start to feel like a leaky, if not fully open, faucet.

The urethra is also unfortunately placed between the clitoris and the vagina. First of all, this means that you practically need to draw a map to communicate effectively with your sexual partner. ("Touch here, caress here, stroke here, but don't touch there.") The urethra is easily irritated, and foreplay can be difficult with somebody who is not at least a little knowledgeable about the placement of our external organs. Also, with all the hands, mouths, and whatever else goes on down there, your urethra sees a lot of bacteria that it could do without.

. . . is bizarre. If you're going to squat in a public bathroom, for God's sake don't spray the toilet seat for the next person who has weak thighs. People have studied different viruses left on toilet seats, and almost every single one was dead within fifteen minutes. If the person right before you sits on the toilet with an open oozing cold sore on the back of her thigh, and you sit down five minutes later, you could possibly get a cold sore in the same place. So you're biggest risk is intermission at the theater where seventy-two women use the toilet in quick succession, but in a normal state of affairs, that toilet seat has been unoccupied for ten minutes. There are those women (for example, the two of us) for whom the odds seem so ridiculous, and who have arthritis (Mom) or are lazy (Liz), for whom squatting is undesirable. One has to estimate these risks at one in one hundred thousand or less. And if you do squat, either wipe off the seat or lift it up so that the next person doesn't have to deal with puddles of your urine.

THE BLADDER

The bladder is also poorly designed, with few muscles to keep it in place. The bottom wall of the bladder is the top wall of the vagina. As goes the vagina, so does the bladder—trauma to one is trauma to the other. Weakness in one is weakness in the other.

THE RECTUM

There is an obsession with bowel function throughout the world, but nowhere is it as pervasive as here in the United States. The bottom wall of the vagina is the same as the top wall of the rectum. The same rules apply as for the shared wall between the vagina and the bladder; injury to one is injury to the other. Rectal problems or infections can directly lead to vaginal infections.

Progesterone, a female hormone (more on this on page 18) can affect bowel function rather easily. It slows things down so we don't have the same peristaltic (i.e. wavelike contractions in our intestines) activity as men.

Let's not go crazy over this. Many women have normal bowel movements daily, while others go two times a week and they're happy. No matter the regularity, the stool should be moist, bulky, and it shouldn't take huge amounts of work, pressure, sweating, straining, and long periods of sitting to get it out. Water is essential for moist bowel function. Fiber is also of paramount importance for keeping the colon healthy. Anything your body can't really digest (think corn) will polish the inside walls of your colon to your healthy advantage.

THE VAGINA

The walls of your vagina are hormone dependent, and, in a functionally mature woman, they are moist from glisteny secretions like the sheen on the surface of an eyeball. This "goo" is made mostly of water and protects the walls of the vagina from abrasion and injury. It's also a recreational lubricant, the importance of which cannot be overstated.

All vaginas are loaded with bacteria, fungi, and viruses. It would be unhealthy if not impossible to try to eradicate these bacteria. They promote vaginal cleanliness enzymatically; by eating debris and fighting with one another they keep the environment in a homeostatic state. Every single vagina has some yeast in it, otherwise known as Candida

No Pockets? Use Your Vagina!

A patient was having an extremely heavy period and was understandably upset. When she came into the office for an exam, I found a tampon. She apologized—she had been bleeding so heavily and was so distracted, she had forgotten. I continued my examination and found three more tampons. In her panic she kept shoving in more tampons to stop the flow of blood. Our point is the vagina is an elastic stretchable thing.

or Monilia. But every vagina also has a natural enemy to yeast—a bacteria called Doderlein's Bacillus or Lactobacillus (the live culture in yogurt). (See page 244 for more on yeast infections.)

EXTERNAL GENITALIA

MONS, LABIA MAJORA, AND CLITORIS

The external genitalia are, in a natural state, covered with hair, as is the mons. Also called "the mound of Venus," this is the fat that covers the pubic bone protecting it from a potentially very painful direct blow. The labia majora are the hair-covered external lips of the vagina. They contain many blood vessels and the mysterious Bartholin's gland. No one knows what the Bartholin's gland does, much like the appendix. Nestled underneath the middle of the pubic bone at the apex of the labia minora, is the clitoris.

LABIA MINORA

At the top of the clitoris, there is a fleshy tissue hood that extends down into two wing shaped appendages called the labia minora. These are hairless, thin, sensitive, and often not symmetrical. A friend in medical school said that he and his friends would check out women in thin

A Word on Waxing Fashions

My days of pelvic exams reveal that there is less and less hair on the labia majora as the years have gone by. The Mohican look, as I call it, is just a strip of hair at the top of the mons—a token remnant. The very popular Brazilian wax denudes almost the entire exterior genitalia of hair. I don't know that there are any health hazards associated with removing your pubic hair, but it sure must hurt. And there are many unfortunate women who, in their dogged pursuit of fashion, have made their genitalia more unsightly with ingrown hairs, pimples, and rashes— a common result of waxing.

I had a patient whose husband would joke about her unusually long labia with his friends and in front of her. I explained that her labia were perfectly normal, but she insisted on having them surgically "corrected." Labiaplasty is a purely cosmetic correction of a real, or in this case, imagined, deformity. There are women with massively abnormal genitalia who never consider changing it, and, as long as they're happy, there is certainly no reason to. By the time this particular patient got the labiaplasty (at her husband's expense), she was divorced.

bathing suits at the beach and guess whether they were "lefties" or a "righties." In retrospect, I think he was lying.

Some labia minora are very pigmented and dark. Some are very long, extending past the labia majora by an inch. Some of them are very asymmetrical, one being much longer than the other. This is all normal. Even so, some women can be very insecure about them, remembering that, in the majority of cases, women don't see or hear about any vaginas, not even their own.

PERINEUM

There are two distances on the pelvic floor that are of some interest. The first is the length of the perineum—the area from the back of the vagina to the rectum. A very short perineum (classified as an inch or less) is of some concern to your obstetrician during childbearing, because no one wants the vagina to rip into the rectum.

The other important distance is from the vaginal opening to the clitoris. This is of more concern to the woman than the doctor, because no matter how close they are, you always think if they were a little closer, life would be so much better. It's never close enough.

* * * * *

DAUGHTER: "So, why gynecology?"

MOTHER: "When I was in medical school, I rotated through all the specialties. I just knew I wanted to be a doctor. And I discovered a few things. Men are the worst patients. They whine, they carry on, they won't get out of bed...."

DAUGHTER: "How come?"

MOTHER: "They don't like being helpless. They don't like being stuck in bed, so they revert to infancy. Don't get me wrong, women can be bitches too, but they complain about auxiliary things. The nurse is bad, the food sucks, blah blah. Men were difficult."

DAUGHTER: "And you had to go to med school to learn that?"

chapter two

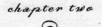

THE PERIOD

I first got my period in a gym bathroom at school when I was about twelve. I pretty much understood what had happened, and my first response was to look at the ceiling and say aloud, "Oh, no." Menstruating signified the end of being bigger and stronger than all the boys, so no more bullying them around. My femininity was tangibly confirmed, and it seemed to me a stain of weakness.

Then I considered how long I could wait before telling my mother. Mom lacks discretion and subtlety when it comes to information pertaining to me. There was a distinct possibility that she'd send out announcements....

Elizabeth Got Her Period!

April 6, 1988

Grade School Gym Class

Basketball

So I told her a month later under the strictest secrecy in the bathroom of a neighborhood Japanese restaurant and made her swear not to tell Dad. Then I imposed a three-year moratorium on period discussions of any kind. Of course, that didn't last.

At least it didn't take long to figure out how to bully the boys around without the benefit of brute strength.

A young woman can get her first period anywhere between ten and sixteen years of age. In general, girls are menstruating earlier than ever before. There are multiple factors that contribute to timing here, and most of them are unknown. Of course, there's a strong hereditary element in just about everything, periods included. Weight is another factor, because fat makes estrogen. Delayed onset of menstruation is rare, but if you haven't bled by age sixteen, see a gynecologist.

YOUR MENSTRUAL CYCLE: A REFRESHER COURSE

At puberty, our complex hormonal trigger system for reproduction spurts to life. Like an old car that takes a few tries to get going, menstruation doesn't always work perfectly from the beginning. First, little flutters of hormonal activity cause secondary sex characteristics to develop. Girls get nipples and pubic and armpit hair. They develop feminine curves. Sometime around then, girls commence menstruation.

The first period happens when the hypothalamus (the most primitive part of the brain) produces gonadotropin releasing hormone (GnRH). This stimulates the pituitary (AKA the master gland) to make gonadotropins, which include follicle stimulating hormone (FSH) and luteinizing hormone (LH). You may remember these from Biology 101. The gonadotropins are released into the bloodstream, stimulating the ovaries to make estrogen and progesterone—the major hormonal players in your reproductive cycle. They stimulate the uterus in a cyclic manner.

Within the ovary, the units of reproduction and hormone production are called follicles. These contain all the essentials (an egg floating in a small sac, the cellular walls of which make estrogen and progesterone) for female reproduction. Technically speaking, a follicle is a tiny fluid-filled cyst. These follicles are pretty much responsible for making us female and the ability to get pregnant. We each have a finite, unique number of these reproduction packages, and cannot make any more (see page 145).

At the beginning of a normal menstrual cycle, FSH interacts with whichever follicles are ripe for stimulation. The one that is the most efficient and responsive surges to the surface of the ovary, leaving the others behind to die off. Every postpubescent, premenopausal day of our lives, tens of follicles prepare to be stimulated by the pituitary and become "the follicle of the month." Very few of these will actually make the journey down the fallopian tubes to the uterus. Sometimes, two or more follicles can head down the road at the same time, and should they meet a couple of lucky sperm, they'll become fraternal twins (or triplets). In any event the majority of follicles develop at suboptimal times in the menstrual cycle, and simply shrivel up and die. So we do not just use one follicle per month, but burn them up at a rate of approximately thirty per day.

For two weeks commencing at the first day of your period, the follicle cells make estrogen. This stimulates the lining of the uterus to get thicker in preparation for a fertilized egg. At ovulation (approximately on day fourteen of the cycle), this hormone-producing "follicle of the month" is big, juicy, and has grown to two to three centimeters in diameter. The estrogen in the bloodstream is high, coursing through the pituitary. At this point the pituitary releases a surge of LH that lasts a day or less. This hormone goes to the ovary, stimulating the rupture of the dominant follicle. Quite literally, it explodes, releasing its precious cargo. This event is ovulation.

The freed egg floats out into the abdominal cavity, hopefully finding its way into the fallopian tube where it may meet a friendly sperm. In

Period Fun Facts

According to Dr. Bruce R. Carr, MD, the average woman in today's industrialized society menstruates 450 times in her life. Compare this to an estimate of only 50 periods for prehistoric women. Even today, in agrarian regions around the world, women only menstruate about 150 times total.

In days of old, doctors thought the ruptured follicle was something other than what we've now determined it is, and they named it *corpus luteum* or "yellow body." It was only in the twentieth century that we realized the empty follicle and the corpus luteum are one in the same.

the meantime, there's a large hole in the ruptured and now empty follicle. The fluid leaks out and, several days later, looks like a yellow patch on the ovary.

The empty follicle (corpus luteum) produces progesterone, in addition to estrogen. Therefore, progesterone is only made between day fourteen of your cycle (ovulation) and your following period. It can only be made if you've ovulated and is essential in the healthy early stages of a pregnancy. At the end of that two-week period, in the absence of a pregnancy, the ovary stops hormone production, the uterine lining that was carefully built during this twenty-eight-day cycle will be shed, and that's your period. Then the whole thing starts over again.

The period itself can last anywhere from two to eight days. Your cycle is the number of days from the first day of your current period to the first day of your next period. The cycle can be as short as twenty-

What Can You do About Heavy Periods?

Some healthy women just happen to have super-heavy periods. The birth control pill can be very helpful, but for extreme cases, there's a new procedure called uterine ablation. Because it applies to such a small percentage of women, it's not very common. Essentially, an extremely hot roller ball is applied to the endometrium, destroying it so that the whole uterine cavity closes and scars over. Lasers and boiling water are also being explored. This is a pretty radical way to cease menstruating, and is obviously not an option for women who want more children.

one days and as long as forty-five. Periods can be very light (wipe and the whole thing is on the toilet paper) or very heavy (two super tampons and a pad every hour). This is a function of "luck." Some people have perfect pitch while others can't carry a tune.

THE BEGINNING

In adolescence, ovulation may not be as efficient or predictable as one might like. When a girl first starts to menstruate, and for some women throughout their lives, the slightest thing can throw her cycle off. A

the period

Some have claimed that menstrual cramps get better after you've had a child. This is probably not true. However, after labor, menstrual cramps aren't comparatively so bad.

final exam, a trip, the flu, a concussion, or any seemingly minor trauma can cause a delay or, conversely, can cause increased bleeding.

Up to the age of about eighteen, irregular periods are quite common. Your body is still working on perfecting the system. Once you're in a menstrual groove, the best way to judge if something is wrong is when it's abnormal. Should anything drastically change—you start bleeding more frequently, or your period lasts twice as long as usual, or you're spotting in between periods and you usually don't—call your doctor.

PMS

Cramps

People have attempted to alleviate menstrual cramps for as long as we've walked upright. Up until the latter half of this century, the medical community had very little to offer. Painkillers were the only option. Women were given opium, heroin, morphine, and aspirin. They used heating pads, hot baths, and electrical stimulators. There was even a brief period when women who complained of cramps were sent to psychiatrists, because menstrual cramps were considered a rejection of one's femininity.

There are many natural ways to treat cramps. Exercise is a very effective treatment, as is a healthy diet. Calcium and Vitamin B6 have been linked to cramp relief as well. It can't hurt to drink plenty of water and get lots of sleep.

For those of you who aren't perfect (like us), you'll be glad to know that science has uncovered the magic of prostaglandins, so called

The essential thing to know about antiprostaglandins is that they will reduce or stop the production of prostaglandins, but will not eliminate those that have already been produced. So, to cure your menstrual cramps with antiprostaglandins, you have to anticipate your period and take them prior to the onset of pain. Of course, if you're already in pain, antiprostaglandins will help, but they take some time to be absorbed and you have to keep taking them to continue alleviating your pain.

because it was first discovered in the prostate gland of a sheep. The Swedes conclusively demonstrated that prostaglandin compounds are always present at the site of pain. These intrepid scientists collected most of Sweden's used tampons and pads, and discovered that women who had severe menstrual cramps had anywhere from twenty to thirty times the amount of prostaglandin in their menstrual blood as women who didn't have cramps. Therefore, antiprostaglandins (aspirin, naproxin, ibuprofen), which were invented for people with joint and bone pain, were ideal for menstrual cramps.

Ultimately, we learned that prostaglandins are produced by the uterine cavity only in a normal ovulating cycle, so if you suppress ovulation, you suppress prostaglandin production. Therefore, 99 percent of women have dramatic relief from cramps on the pill. Systemic contraception also eliminates the hormonal fluctuations that go along with a period, the premenstrual breast pain, etc.

There is no direct link between the amount you bleed and your cramps. However, if you tend to have clottier periods, you will tend to have worse cramps because your uterus needs to contract harder and your cervix needs to dilate to allow the clumps of blood to pass. Because the pill contains both estrogen and progesterone, the lining of your uterus never gets the chance to build up and get as thick as when

the period

17

Anemia with the period can be a very bad cycle. When you're anemic, your blood is more watery, which means that you bleed more because the blood flows more readily. So one of the main causes of heavy periods is anemia, which is made worse by your heavy periods, and this cycle can continue until your hemoglobin is very low and you're at the risk of shock. In this state, you have no safety margin should you suffer an unexpected trauma.

your body is producing estrogen alone (at the outset of a normal cycle). The pill reduces the volume of blood and is therefore an excellent treatment for women who are anemic due to their period.

Mood

Recapping, briefly, we make estrogen alone for the first half of the ovulating cycle. From the middle of the cycle until the next period, your body produces progesterone and estrogen together. Progesterone production increases up until you get your period. You may have noticed that the rising quantity of this particular hormone parallels the increasing severity of a complex of symptoms called *premenstrual syndrome* (PMS). Presently, the politically correct term in the medical community is premenstrual dysphoric disorder (PMDD), which means your doctor may call PMS PMDD. Call it what you like.

If you've ever seen a Mydol commercial, then you know that the symptoms of PMS can include headaches, irritability, depression, crying jags, severe breast pain, abdominal distension, backache, and weight gain. To spin it positively, the second half of the cycle is about making things good for the potential baby on the way; our primitive brain considers every ovulation a chance at a pregnancy. Progesterone stimulates our breasts to get ready to produce milk. Progesterone is mildly sedating, so we can be a little sleepy right before our periods.

Progesterone is a smooth muscle (generally speaking, smooth muscles are involuntary) relaxant, so it can cause the intestinal tract to relax and fill with gas and solid waste. And some women just don't do well emotionally. They pick fights, they're irritable, nasty, and they cry easily.

PMS exists. It's real, and it's complicated. If you had a joint meeting with psychologists, endocrinologists, and gynecologists, they would all agree that it's a multifaceted issue. Primarily, PMS is about hormones, but it is also inextricably tied to our physical surroundings and what's going on in our lives. PMS is usually not so bad on honeymoons, but it's terrible during a divorce. PMS is fine while you're on vacation but is awful when you have a job you hate. So when you're down, PMS makes it worse. When you're up, it doesn't seem to be such a problem.

PMS Theories

Researchers have demonstrated that female prison inmates are much more likely to commit a violent crime premenstrually than postmenstrually. Mary Dalton, a British doctor and self-proclaimed PMS expert, asserts that PMS problems arise from an imbalance between progesterone and estrogen and that the appropriate treatment is more progesterone. She has testified at murder trials, stating that premenstrual rage caused the defendants to commit their crimes, and she could ameliorate their problems with hormones, which, sadly, doesn't seem to be the case. This avenue has been a total dead end. All efforts in the sixties, seventies, and eighties to give additional progesterone premenstrually have not changed anything.

Health food stores are rife with home remedies, many of which claim to help with PMS. There are always new herbs and potions being touted as the next, best, "natural" PMS cure. Most recently, Evening Primrose Oil was conclusively debunked as a treatment strategy. This doesn't mean you have to lose hope in a holistic cure, but none have been clinically proven.

We know that progesterone causes water retention, so another theory is that cerebral edema (brain swelling) causes you to get a little

squirrelly. Some women have benefited from low-salt diets premenstrually and natural diuretics. Lots of water, parsley, asparagus, fruits,
and vegetables in general should help keep you from becoming too ede-
matous. If you can document a three to five pound weight gain the
week before your period, you might benefit from medical diuretics.
Ask your doctor about them.

Our brains make their own endorphins, also known as the "tran-
quilizer within." Some studies have suggested that we make fewer
endorphins premenstrually, and therefore, it's not that we're more irritable, we're just less tranquil. If this theory sounds good to you, then
try Vitamin B6. It's a natural diuretic, so it combats the edema. It also is
an essential enzyme in endorphin production, so B6 has been shown to
help with mood swings, depression, anxiety, and irritability. Vitamin E
is another option; some of my patients claim great relief from their
symptoms, though the medical community has little explanation of
why this is so. You can take all of these vitamins as pills, or find them in
foods such as leafy green vegetables.

One study (probably conducted by Dr. Atkins) suggested we
might have a premenstrual intolerance to carbohydrates; i.e. our glu-
cose tolerance tests can be slightly abnormal the week before our periods, and totally normal the week afterward. We all know the urge for
chocolate and candy premenstrually. This is probably cultural—we've
learned to associate yummy chocolate with comfort and indulgence.
When you eat a candy bar, your blood sugar goes up and you get
sleepy. Then your blood sugar tumbles and you get a little irritable, so
you have another candy bar (this cycle doesn't just apply to PMS).
Thus you have constant fluctuations in mood mirroring your fluctuations in blood sugar. You should stick with vegetables, fruit, and whole
grains for any sweets you need (we wish we were kidding). Recent
studies also suggest that high doses of calcium (1000 milligrams per
day) may help to improve your premenstrual mood.

One very strange study suggested that women with severe hospi-
talizable PMS were sexually abused as children. The psychiatric theory
here is that PMS may be a time when we are very libidinous (i.e. horny)

but when you're sexually dysfunctional, horniness might make you irritable. For those of us that are sexually functional, it's ironic that we pick more fights with our sexual partners at a time when we most want what they have to offer.

Everyone knows that caffeine is an irritant. It jangles the nerves and makes our hands jittery. You may want to avoid indulging in too much coffee the week before your period, because it will only add fuel to the fire. Regardless of PMS, if you are a major caffeine consumer (more than three large cups of coffee per day or the equivalent), then you should probably cut back anyway. Too much caffeine clearly causes mildly annoying symptoms (jumpiness), but can also lead to very significant problems (e.g. negative cardiovascular events).

As for period-specific medications, these are usually a combination diuretic (for the swelling) and aspirin (for the discomfort) so they're hardly a breakthrough cure.

All of these theories probably contain a grain of truth, but there is no magic formula. If you feel that the quality of your life is jeopardized premenstrually, is secondary to real physical causes, and you've tried all the natural approaches, the most current treatment option is Serafim (Prozac with a different name). Antianxiety and antidepression pills have been successfully prescribed for PMS. This may sound extreme, but many women extol the virtues of an occasional antidepressant to prevent a full day of inexplicable crying in bed. And there's the birth control pill, which has always been at the forefront of PMS prevention.

MENSTRUAL IRREGULARITIES

DUB—Dysfunctional Uterine Bleeding, Oligomenorrhea, Amenorrhea

Dysfunctional uterine bleeding (DUB) is abnormal, increased vaginal bleeding for which no physical cause can be found. This includes spotting between periods, prolonged periods, and short cycles. Oligomenorrhea is when the patient has her periods less frequently than normal, and amenorrhea is when she doesn't get her period at all.

I often see patients who are clearly not getting their period because they are way too thin. I have a patient who has vaginal bleeding every time she has a fight with her mother. I see another woman who bleeds when a relative is in the hospital or every time she goes to a funeral. You don't need to be a doctor to suspect that these women might benefit from therapy. As their physician, I suggest, plead, and nag them about therapy and sometimes this works. They get better, eat more, address their latent emotional issues, and resume having their period regularly and naturally. However, this is the exception to the rule. Most gynecological patients do not hearken to unsolicited therapy referrals.

As with ovarian growths (see page 192) the most essential directive for the physician is to determine that there are, in fact, no physical or hormonal causes for the patient's abnormal menstrual cycles, including pregnancy, hormonal imbalances of the thyroid, pituitary and ovaries, structural abnormalities, etc. When everything has been tested and nothing wrong is found, the doctor is then concerned with the long-term implications of the situation. All prolonged menstrual irregularities that are without physical cause contribute to endometrial disease (cancer).

Treatment
Menstrual irregularities without physical cause are attributed to hypothalamic dysfunction, which can be tied to physical (e.g. a concussion) or emotional stress (e.g. a final exam). There are several ways to address this medically. The easiest is to prescribe the birth control pill, which provides measured amounts of both progesterone and estrogen (see page 73 for more on the pill). Progesterone is another option. Given for ten to twelve days at a time, it mimicks but does not provoke ovulation. Within seven days of the last dose of progesterone, the

patient will have a bleeding episode. So the progesterone worked with her own estrogen production, built up and shed the lining, protecting her from endometrial overstimulation. More complicated is to prescribe pituitary hormones (FSH and LH) to stimulate the follicle, synthetically triggering ovulation.

The other way to handle irregular periods is to address the root problem, though this generally goes beyond the conventional gynecologist's role. Often, women do not get their period for reasons that are directly linked to their behavior (e.g. not eating) or a particular emotional stressor that they have not fully addressed. Trying to encourage these women to get appropriate help can be extremely difficult, as ther-

A Word About Eating Disorders

Weight loss is currently the best-known cause of a lost period. The hypothalamus controls your body by producing hormones called "releasing factors;" these influence the pituitary to make all the hormones in the body. When the hypothalamus sees you wasting away, it says, "Well, let's not get pregnant now. Let's not lose any blood. Let's stop this nonessential function so that we can preserve our scant nutrition for vital organs." If you are voluntarily not eating or overexercising, your fat to muscle ratio may fall below healthy levels, which will turn off your body's production of follicle-stimulating hormone. The ovary will independently make small amounts of estrogen. This means that a few follicles grow a little and make a little hormone. Then they die because they haven't been stimulated enough to continue growing, and there is no lutenizing hormone to trigger ovulation. This leads to polycystic ovaries and an overstimulated uterus, because you're not making any of the counterbalancing progesterone (since you're not ovulating) and therefore not shedding the uterine lining each month. Eventually, this could contribute to uterine cancer. Needless to say, if undereating and overexercising are your modus operandi, you're tampering with your long-term reproductive health.

apy is a far lengthier, more costly, emotionally treacherous route than simply taking some pills.

There are no cut-and-dry guidelines for maintaining a regular period; some women marathon runners have no trouble with their cycle, while other women start running a few miles each day and they stop bleeding. Some women run international conglomerates and can set their watch by their period, while others throw their cycle off over the holidays.

YOUR PERIOD AFFECTS YOUR VAGINA

In the first half of your cycle estrogen stimulates your vagina and cervix to make a secretion that's very similar to raw egg white. It's clear, elastic, and has a high salt content—a hospitable environment for sperm. It's a very swimmable medium, which helps them maneuver the difficult passage through the cervix. This discharge increases in quantity until you ovulate.

Once you've ovulated (in the middle of the cycle), progesterone is added to the hormonal soup of your body. The progesterone-estrogen combination will change your vaginal discharge. It becomes creamy and sticky, thereby plugging up the cervix and preventing sperm from getting in. Your body doesn't want any more sperm in your uterus, because theoretically the fertilized egg may be wending its way down the fallopian tube. The last thing you want is a crowd of sperm making it difficult for the new embryo to implant in the uterine lining.

This creamy discharge gets heavier as you approach your period and can be a bit gamey (ergo that fishy reputation). Secretions are the heaviest at the end of the cycle. Then you menstruate and the whole thing starts all over again.

As this is all going on, from the first day of your cycle to your next period, the PH (a measure of acidity) drops consistently and the environment in your vagina becomes more acidic. Acid is friendly to yeast, which is why you may notice your vagina gets itchier the closer you are to your period. It's common, and almost always goes away when the PH in your vagina rises with menstruation.

Toxic Shock Syndrome (TSS) made headlines when it struck a handful of women in North America. They had been using highly absorbent tampons, which are probably a little more abrasive to the vaginal walls, and they had staph aureus in their vaginas. The mild hysteria associated with this newly labeled condition made women phobic about tampons.

TOXIC SHOCK SYNDROME

TSS is defined as the presence of staphylococcus aureus toxins in the bloodstream, leading to high fever, vascular collapse, and in some cases, death. To even possibly be struck by this syndrome, you have to have had a break in the integument (the surface of the body: skin, nose, vagina), which is the inroad for the bacteria. And the bacteria must be present at the site and time of breakage.

The vast majority of TSS has nothing to do with tampons or vaginas. Men get it. Postmenopausal women get it. And if you have forgotten a tampon and left it in for longer than you would have liked, the odds of your getting TSS remain very close to zero.

Basic symptoms of TSS include a temperature of at least 103 degrees Farenheit and a reddish rash all over your body, most likely on your hands and feet. Feeling a little achy is not Toxic Shock Syndrome. If you are really nervous about it, ask your gynecologist to take a vaginal culture. If there's no staph aureus in your vagina, then you probably won't get TSS. If you do have it, then you should take antibiotics and get rid of it so that you're not at risk and can stop worrying.

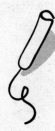

Some women are still fearful of tampons, both because of TSS and due to a distaste for touching their vaginas. I've had women come into my office so that I can go after a tampon, because they don't want to put their own fingers inside their vagina. The whole point of this book is to become more comfortable with your vagina and all its idiosyncrasies. Touch it, test it out, and, if you've been avoiding them because your vagina grosses you out, give tampons a test drive. It might change your life.

TAMPONS VS. PADS

Tampons are not really for the lightest days of your period, when you're barely bleeding, because they sop up your natural secretions. This irritates the vagina, which likes to be moist. If the tampon hurts a little coming out, and it's still mostly dry, that's a tampon you shouldn't have put in in the first place.

Women who wear pads probably have their own set of problems. It's irritating to the external genitalia. With all due respect to sanitary napkins and the women who love them, they can ride up, they can get stuck between the cheeks of your buttocks, and it's got to be annoying having a foreign body in your underwear all the time. For obvious reasons, pads are not an attractive option for athletic women—the sweat and movement can dislodge them from your underwear.

Some women use tampons during the day and pads at night. If it makes you happy, sure. If you're having moderate to heavy bleeding (you saturate a tampon every two to three hours), then tampons are perfectly safe. If it's scant, and you can barely see any blood on the tip of the tampon, then you should probably stick with minipads. Or use the skinniest tampon you can find.

Tampons for Teens

I had a mother bring her fourteen-year-old daughter to see me. The mother was clearly agitated, and both women were reluctant to tell me why they were in my office. Finally, the mother blurts out, "Go ahead. Go ahead and tell her." Turns out the girl wanted to learn how to use tampons, and the mother felt they were dangerous and unhealthy. I assured her that this was not the case, took her daughter into the exam room, got out a big mirror, and showed her where they went (she'd been focusing on the wrong hole). It was very exciting for her, and she felt like a real adult when she left my office, confident with using tampons.

CULTURAL HISTORY

Many religions state that menstruation is unclean. It's safe to say that this misinformation is promoted in an effort to emphasize vaginal intercourse during the more fertile period, thereby increasing the population. Circulating the belief that menstrual fluid is filthy works in societies where proliferation is the primary objective. There is no truth to this whatsoever—it's perfectly fine to have sex during your period. The major risk is to your sheets. And I wish they would choose a word other than *unclean*. There is nothing unclean about menstruation or any normal bodily fluid, like saliva or tears.

Things Change

Most women have relatively the same period from cycle to cycle. It's on the macro level that you notice chances. Your period could easily be different (longer, shorter, more or less disruptive) at forty than it was at twenty.

* * * * *

DAUGHTER: "Do you get menstrual cramps?"

MOTHER: "No. Do you?"

DAUGHTER: "No."

MOTHER: "I went through labor, though."

DAUGHTER: "Thanks, Mom. You're the best."

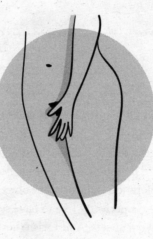

chapter three

THE GYNECOLOGIST

Going to the gynecologist for the first time was a little dif-. ferent for me than for most girls. I was:

A) going to my mother's office,
B) entirely familiar with the staff,
C) very friendly with my doctor who was my mother's partner at the time, and
D) pretty sure that I could handle whatever they were going to throw at me.

And still, I must have been pretty nervous in a quiet, protective sort of way, because I can't remember a thing about it.

The American College of OB-GYN's most recent standards suggest that your first visit to a gynecologist be no more than three years after your first sexual encounter, and thereafter you should see your doctor once a year. I disagree. Ideally, women should go see a gynecologist when they're thinking about becoming sexually active, so that they can discuss all of their personal issues and concerns with their doctor, including, but not limited to, contraception. Failing that, I recommend women get to the gynecologist between the ages of eighteen and twenty-one.

Ninety percent of gynecology has to do with sex. You're either trying not to catch something, checking if you did catch something, preventing pregnancy, seeing if you are pregnant, trying to have a baby, having a baby, or not having a baby. Therefore, most of the issues the OB-GYN faces do not present themselves in a woman who's never been

It's impossible to speak for all gynecologists everywhere. I've tried to consider the possible variations on a gynecological visit, but this is mostly an overview of what I do with my patients. For example, in this harried HMO environment, there is a premium on a doctor's time and she may elect not to do breast exams, so you might consider inquiring about them.

sexually active. But there are exceptions: tumors, cysts that get out of control, vaginal infections, and abnormalities in menstruation regardless of sexual activity. It behooves an adult woman to have an annual visit with her doctor.

THE BLOW-BY-BLOW

THE PREAMBLE

Your trip to the gynecologist should be extremely anticlimactic. The anticipation is almost always much worse than anything that's going to happen to you at the doctor's office. Of course, there are gynecologists who might be a teeny bit insensitive, and you may not have much of a choice. If not, buck up and bear it until you can get another doctor. It's your health, after all.

The first order of business will be your history, which you generally provide on a form that you fill out yourself with medical, obstetrical, and gynecological information on it (e.g. how many times have you been pregnant, have you had any abortions, family histories of cancer, surgical history, medical history, allergies, etc.). After you have filled in all your information, you should meet the doctor in her consultation room.

At this point, a good doctor will peruse your history and extrapolate from it. She should ask questions, try to clarify what you wrote down, make sure nothing has been overlooked, and then address your questions, concerns, and any present symptoms.

Then you will be escorted into an examining room where you disrobe. You could take this opportunity to detour to the ladies room to pee, as a full bladder makes the pelvic exam uncomfortable and less accurate. From the doctor's point of view, giving a gynecological exam through a full bladder is like feeling a plum through a balloon. Additionally, you should try not to go to your gynecologist when you are menstruating. It makes your Pap smear inaccurate.

Some doctors will take a urine sample. At my office, I only take urine from pregnant patients, or if there is a history of bladder or kidney problems, or current symptoms of infection. While I think routine samples are excessive, it certainly does no harm, and occasionally the doctor might catch something she might have otherwise missed.

While you wait for the doctor in the exam room, a nurse or physician's assistant may take your blood pressure and weigh you. The blood pressure is essential. Cardiovascular disease, which includes hypertension, kills more women in this country than the next fourteen causes of death put together. Taking a blood pressure is a simple, noninvasive, critical test that should be done at any and every doctor's visit (perhaps not the dermatologist).

Getting weighed isn't fun for most people, and some of my patients refuse. Look, no one is judging your weight. No one's going to yell at you. No one wants to embarrass you. But, if you're lucky,

---

Unexpected Medical Histories

When I was first starting out, a new patient came in. On her medical history she had written "therapist" as her occupation. Now, these were the early days so I had a lot of time on my hands. As I was making conversation, I asked, "Are you a Freudian or Jungian therapist?" She responded, "I'm a hooker." I said, "I guess that's a type of therapy." "I think so," said she.

Unless you've been living under a rock, you know that being overweight is bad for your health. Diabetes, heart disease, joint problems, and a hundred other health issues are tied to fat. However, women who weigh more than 150 pounds are far less likely to develop osteoporosis, because their bones remain strong carrying around the additional weight. So that's one good thing to think about while you try to lose weight. If you're lighter, lift weights for comparable benefit to your bones.

you're building a relationship with a doctor that could last twenty years or more. And you'll be the first person to say at each annual visit, "What did I weigh last year?" It will annoy you more than your doctor to have to say, "I'm sorry, you refused to be weighed." This way, we can all tell early signs of gradual weight gain. It's much easier to hear that you've gained five pounds than fifty. If you really hate to see the numbers, step on the scale and close your eyes. Finally, the nurse may measure your height if you are older. Loss of height is an early sign of bone loss.

ENTER THE DOCTOR . . .

If the nurse is smart, she'll hand you a magazine while you wait for your doctor to show up. She should be there within thirty seconds, but try to remember there are often good reasons why this doesn't happen. It is nerve-wracking to wait naked in an examining room for the doctor to perform that horrible thing with the clamps and spoons and instruments. It's not intentional. Read *People*.

So the doctor comes in and may, on a first visit, listen to your heart and your lungs, and/or feel your neck to check if your thyroid is swollen, and/or look down your throat. These are things that may also be done by a general medical physician.

Then there's the breast exam. The doctor will first look at your breasts. She is looking for skin changes, a bulge, a dimple, asymmetry (which is extremely normal and common, but dramatic asymmetry can suggest a problem), or redness. She may ask you to shrug your shoulders or lift your arms to make sure that your breasts move with your arms and are not fixed to your chest wall. She will examine your breasts sitting up, with one hand underneath and one hand on top of each breast, covering the entire breast area. She will gently squeeze the nipple to make sure there is no discharge.

Then you lie down and she will examine you again, sometimes with a pillow under your shoulder blade and with the arm of the examined breast over your head. She should examine up into your armpit for swollen glands, making sure that every square inch of breast tissue is covered. In general, the sitting exam is for superficial lumps, and the lying-down exam is for breast conditions or lesions that are closer to the chest wall.

Now that you're lying down, it's time for an abdominal exam. Your doctor will take her hands and palpate (touch) all four quadrants of the abdomen, digging under the ribs on both sides. This is to check for any swelling, tenderness, growths, or masses.

LET THE GAMES BEGIN

Then there are the stirrups. I don't know why we call them stirrups. If you have a good imagination, they look like stirrups on a saddle, but you don't put your feet through the holes. Your heel rests in the curve of the stirrup as you lie down and then you let your knees fall apart. Then the doctor will position you by pulling your hips down to the edge of the table to accommodate the speculum.

The speculum. The dreaded speculum. It's generally metal, but there are also disposable plastic models. It has usually been sterilized but is not kept in sterile packaging. Just like a tampon, there is no need for it to be perfectly sterile, but it has to be clean. The speculum is a simple modification of two spoons. If you think of the vagina as a stretchable tube, two inserted spoons spread apart are a good way to see

··

The speculum was invented by J. Marion Sims, who also founded the New York Infirmary and is called the "Father of American Gynecology." He wasn't a very nice man, and most historians will back us up on that. He pioneered gynecological surgery by practicing on slaves, without consent and certainly without the benefit of anesthesia. His statue is in Central Park, so feel free to go and throw things at it.

··

the top of the vagina, where the cervix is, as well as the walls of the vagina. This is how your doctor can evaluate vaginal secretions for possible infections, as well as look for growths like polyps, abrasions, and irritations.

I promise a speculum exam does not hurt. There are certainly patients who have very unpleasant stories about rough or clumsy doctors. Surely, a cold speculum can be quite a surprise. It's a technique doctors learn through practice, so if your doctor hasn't done a lot of them, she may be a little awkward and it might be uncomfortable. In the hands of an experienced gynecologist, a speculum should be no more painful than an ear exam.

At this point, the doctor will do a Pap smear. This involves a small brush or spatula that the physician uses to obtain exfoliated cells from the cervix and, in the case of a good Pap smear, the cervical canal. A Pap smear can twinge a little, but the majority of patients aren't that bothered. It is not uncommon to have a little bleeding after a Pap smear. This is something you can completely ignore. The Pap concept is that free-floating cells can tell us about the tissue they came from. So if you have a free-floating cell that looks abnormal, you can say with some confidence that that cell came from cancerous or precancerous tissue. The same concept is applied to smears taken from the cheek, nose, or rectum, but its primarily applied to diagnose cervical problems (see page 235 for more Pap smear information).

Following the removal of the speculum, equally important if not more so, is the bimanual examination. Your doctor will insert one or two fingers (which should be lubricated with KY Jelly) in your vagina, and place her other hand on your abdomen wall. The uterus and ovaries can be felt between those two hands, so that the doctor can feel if the uterus is enlarged, bumpy, or tender. She can wiggle the cervix; if it hurts, that may indicate irritation or inflammation. This is where the empty bladder comes in handy. Your bladder rests right on your uterus, so if you have a full bladder your doctor will have a hard time feeling through all that liquid. I ask people to pee if this is the case.

Additionally, I've asked patients to come back after a bowel movement. Constipation can feel like a very large ovarian tumor. Your colon is on both sides, so it's not uncommon for someone who hasn't had a bowel movement that day to feel to the physician as if they have a pelvic mass.

Outside of urine and stool, it's important to try and relax your abdominal wall. The idea is to make your belly as soft as you can, because if you make a muscle, your doctor will have to push through it. This is both uncomfortable and inaccurate. If it is your first visit, and you have no symptoms, your physician may let this go. It is of paramount importance to have a patient who is not unhappy or fearful about her next visit, and is readily willing to see a gynecologist in the future.

And that's the sum of it. There's nothing to fear, except the reprimanding you can count on if you stay away for more than a year. In the best of all worlds, you should establish a good relationship with your doctor, which can last for decades. Not only will this improve the quality of your healthcare because she knows you, but you'll be more likely to go regularly.

* * * * *

MOTHER: "You don't remember anything about your first time?"

DAUGHTER: "Nope."

MOTHER: "Do you remember anything about any of your trips to the gynecologist?"

DAUGHTER: "Not really. Actually, it's been a while..."

MOTHER: "Me too."

DAUGHTER: "Do as I say..."

MOTHER: "And not as I do."

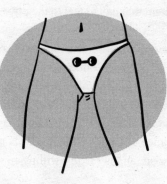

chapter four

MAINTENANCE

Thanks to the douching industry, we now have a euphemism for a smelly crotch. However, that "not-so-fresh feeling," is not something that you should go to war over. Not only are odor and moistness appropriate for your vagina, but, as with so many things, when you try to fine-tune something that was fine to begin with, you risk ending up far worse off than where you started.

Like most businesses, the douche people have worked hard to make us all feel insecure about our vaginas to the point where we need to do something about them, which may include buying their product. The best thing to do here is not let them make you insecure in the first place. Forget douching—it's unnecessary and can create problems where there were none.

Instead, do the *simple* and *easy* things in this chapter to maintain your vaginal health. The smallest effort today could produce significant results as you get older and your body becomes less able to bounce back from life's little road bumps.

OVARIES

It might seem like there's not much going on with your ovaries—they're chock-full of follicles in a state of suspended animation waiting to grow. And yet in other ways there's always a follicle growing, an egg waiting to leave, or a cyst forming. The birth control pill is the number one helpful thing you can do for your ovaries because the pill prevents cell division, lessening the chance of abnormal growths and cancer.

The ovaries are somewhat sensitive to radiation. That's why when you go to the dentist and get an X ray, she puts a lead shield over your abdomen. Your ovaries contain your only reproductive opportunities, and they're precious and finite. So perhaps Chernobyl is not a good place to go on vacation. If you should visit a friend in an ICU at the hospital and they're taking an X ray in the next bed, get out of the room.

There are other, more likely, ways we get radiated. If you go to an emergency room with a sprained ankle or a bad cold, you'll probably be X-rayed. Someone on the hospital staff should ask when your last period was, to ensure that you're not pregnant. You're exposed to radiation when you sit close to a TV or computer monitor. The further away you are from it, the less detectable the radiation is. So your mother was right, don't sit too close to the television. Try not to press your ovaries to the microwave door. You are radiated when you go on a plane. They estimate that a cross-continental flight is the equivalent radiation of a mammogram.

These are just things to be aware of, not rules to live by. Don't cancel your vacation to Europe to avoid the radiation.

THE TUBES

There's not much you can do on a day-to-day basis to maintain fallopian tube health, except avoid unprotected sex. At the hands of gonorrhea, chlamydia, and other pelvic infections, your tubes can sustain irrevocable damage.

THE UTERUS

In an unpregnant state, the uterus sits like an innocuous dried plum waiting for its chance to ripen.

CERVIX

The cervix is very vulnerable to infection (see page 234), so, again, it comés down to knowing what you're putting in your vagina. Make sure he has a condom on. Cervical disease is virtually unheard of in a celibate woman. Almost everything that happens to the cervix is related to sex. Pick your playmates carefully.

THE BLADDER

The bladder is a pain in the neck, but think what life would be like if we didn't have one. It's not built like steel. Hell, it's not even built well. Luckily, we have some tactics to help make your bladder become all it can be.

Please please PLEASE do your Kegel's exercises. These are vaginal exercises that counteract the years of gravitational pull on our bladders. Every woman should do these exercises every day forever. When you urinate, stop the stream. Slow it down if you can't stop it. Do this at least once a day. This maintains the muscles that close your urethra.

Doing your Kegel's while peeing is an easy way to remember, but you can really do them anytime. Think about it this way, when you're moving your bowels, the first half you push, then the second half you squeeze. When you make this muscle, it should feel as if you're pulling your rectum towards your vagina. Squeeze, hold it for three seconds, then relax. Do it anytime, stopped at a red light, waiting at the dentist's office, whenever. It's the easiest exercise we can think of. It increases vaginal muscle tone, and the strength of your whole perineum. It is even more important after childbirth, but regardless, nothing can battle eighty years of gravity, coughing, and laughing like consistent Kegeling. Also,

maintenance

Kegel's in a Nutshell

PEE – stop – PEE – stop – PEE – stop – PEE (aaaah)

You're wandering in the forest. On your right along your little garden path is a stagnant, murky pond. A green film coats the surface, dotted only by the occasional slimy toad. Large, nasty looking bugs skim the muck. On your left is a babbling brook, with crystal clear water trickling over smooth, clean rocks. It's delicious, healthy, and refreshing. Which do you want to be? The stagnant pond or the babbling brook? The path to the brook is water. Drink water in copious amounts and everything keeps flowing.

DAUGHTER: "You don't ever drink water."

MOTHER: "Do what I say."

DAUGHTER: "And not what you do."

MOTHER: "Right."

DAUGHTER: "Because coffee doesn't get you to the babbling brook."

MOTHER: "All right already."

as if you needed yet another reason to do this essential exercise, guys really like it when you Kegel (without the peeing) during sex.

URETHRA

The urethra just wants to be left alone.

VAGINA

Every time you tamper with your vagina's natural environment, you risk destabilizing an entire ecosystem. Douching causes more problems than it's worth. Antiseptic douches will kill the normal healthy bacteria that prevent pathogenic bacteria from gaining a toehold in your vagina. A vinegar douche is astringent (like sucking on a lemon) and dries up natural secretions, making intercourse or any vaginal visitation more traumatic. A douche will also tamper with the PH in your vagina, encouraging certain natural inhabitants to grow beyond their normal proportions resulting in clinical symptoms. And, remember, there can always be a rebound effect. Your body could respond to a vinegar douche with heaps of extra secretions.

With that in mind, there are certain women who, no matter what we say, simply must meddle with the status quo. In fairness, some vaginas are wetter than others. This tends to be a Mediterranean problem (or advantage, depending on your point of view) along with moustaches and hearty appetites. But if you feel that you have an excessive amount of vaginal secretions or if you just sweat more down there than you're comfortable with, limit yourself to a once-per-month, postmenstrual, astringent (e.g. vinegar) douche. But this is only if you absolutely insist on douching at all.

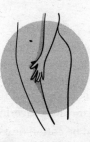

A Word about the Smell

....

Make no mistake, all crotches smell at the end of the day. The more nerve-wracking or active the day, the more we smell. There's nothing better than a nice shower, but some women feel that external deodorant sprays specifically intended for your crotch are a reasonable alternative when a shower is inconvenient. These are certainly not obligatory or suggested, but are also not harmful, and may help you feel less self-conscious if you feel you're particularly smelly. You can also use scented tampons to no ill effect, but only when you have your period and never in between. And however offensively you think you smell, it's not nearly as bad as you think.

....

Whatever you do, do not use tampons for everyday vaginal secretions. Therein lies disaster. Approximately one patient per month admits they wear tampons twenty-four hours a day, seven days a week, fifty-two weeks a year. Tampons are designed for absorption and will suck up anything in their path. They can dehydrate the walls of your vagina and will push your symptoms into overdrive as your vagina tries to keep pace with the unanticipated dryness by making more and more secretions. The tampons can irritate the walls of the vagina, causing abrasions and chafing. Any foreign body in your vagina will attract more bacteria. This is an altogether untenable biological situation for your vagina. Like a drug dependency, it can take weeks to months to correct.

PANTY CHOICES AND YOUR VAGINA

I have no comment on thongs. Okay, I have a few comments. They look terribly uncomfortable to me. I am told, "Wear them once and you'll never go back." But the area covering the vaginal opening and the external genitalia should be cotton or cotton-crotched, to allow air in and absorb moisture. Synthetic fibers are airtight, and therefore highly undesirable for direct contact with your vagina. It's been proven that the temperature at the vaginal opening is higher when you wear synthetic fibers, promoting fungus. Also, the material creates an oil slick of sorts, which will chafe and irritate.

Another thing I don't understand is the panty liner. I know that every once in a while there are secretions that can stain your panties. Weigh how much it costs to replace your panties a little more frequently versus the discomfort, irritation, and itching of a pad. And of course, millions of synthetic fiber pads thrown away each day are hardly helping the earth. It seems like a no-brainer to me, and yet many women choose everyday minipads.

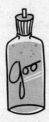

DID YOU THINK WE WEREN'T GOING TO TALK ABOUT SEX AND YOUR VAGINA?

We are still harvesting the fruits of a sexual revolution, so we are using our vaginas a whole lot more than we used to. Friction in the vagina, like sandpaper, will irritate the walls and cause the temperature to rise. So, if you're going to have more intercourse than your body can make lubrication for (e.g. your boyfriend's back from the oil rig and the mind is willing but the body isn't able to keep up), use artificial goo. It will help protect your tissues from damage and your bladder from infection.

Another thing to consider when you're about to enjoy the throes of a whole lot of passion is that every thrust of the penis pushes bacteria up from the urethral opening into the bladder. Remember, while there is plenty of normal, healthy bacteria in the vagina, there should be no bacteria in your bladder. A dry vagina exacerbates the situation and is, incidentally, no fun. As you irritate your vagina, you're also pushing bacteria up towards the bladder. And the next day, you wonder why it burns when you urinate.

Try not to clump up on sex. A sudden upswing in activity can cause bladder infections (AKA Honeymoon Cystitis), vaginal infections, and irritations. You're better off having sex every night than just three times

Working out Your Vagina

To maintain vaginal muscle tone, after multiple kids for example, you can purchase heavy metal balls to carry around in your vagina. It's a constant passive workout. Conversely, there are dilaters if you feel you're too tight.

You may be wondering why prostitutes don't have constant bladder infections. My theory is that "Johns" don't exactly hold out and aim to satisfy their hooker, so the (lucky?) women have as much friction on one long night of work as a honeymooner's lightest evening. They're also professionals; so their bodies have grown accustomed to activity that would cause problems for any amateur.

on Saturday. This works really well in theory, but people live in different cities, meet on weekends, are busy working, etc. So we understand if you simply must have a lot of sex on Sunday, but drink more water. Urinate before and after intercourse. Before prevents the full bladder from bombardment by the thrusting penis. Peeing afterwards flushes out the bacteria that were thrust up there by coitus. We can't say it enough—lubricate or you're going to inflame the entire area.

How much sex is too much? We can't say. It depends on age, lubrication, angle, experience, duration, etc. Find what you're comfortable with and try not to push your body too hard.

When it comes to bladder infections, cranberry juice is not a myth. It contains Hippuric acid, which prevents bacteria from multiplying. However, it doesn't kill the bacteria that are already there. So if you feel burning when you urinate, drink as much cranberry juice as possible as soon as possible, which will increase your chances of nipping the problem in the bud. If you continue to have these symptoms for more than twelve hours, it's time to call your doctor.

RECTUM

Around the rectal opening is a plexus of hemorrhoidal veins. When you push hard they will swell, and a swollen hemorrhoidal vein is (you guessed it) a hemorrhoid. Constipated people will get hemorrhoids. People who have diarrhea will get hemorrhoids, not from pushing hard

@vaginas

but pushing frequently. And people who alternate between the diarrhea and the constipation are really in trouble. This is the hallmark of Irritable Bowel Syndrome.

The rectal opening is a lens. When it hits a critical diameter, the skin will split. Large, rocky stools can cause an anal fissure, i.e. a chronic tear in the rim of your anus. This is harder to fix than the perineal fissure (see page 47), because while you can abstain from sex (we promise), you have to have bowel movements. As soon as it starts to get better, it's time to take another dump. This is best to prevent. You want a bulky, moist stool.

Whole grains, fiber, cellulose—stuff that you really don't digest into your blood stream, but rather extract the good stuff and pass it into your intestines—are essential components of a bulky stool. Eat salads, celery greens, whole fruits, whole grains, etc.

Water is also an essential component of healthy bowel movements. Your stool is your last reservoir for moisture. If you are dehydrated, the body will extract every molecule of H_2O in your colon just to maintain bodily function. So by the time you're passing that stool, it's like a rock, with corners and angles.

The Researcher Who Went Where We Probably Would Not

There was a study about the link between diet and, well, shit. A researcher went to an area in Africa where people ate very poorly processed grains that even had some dirt mixed in. He followed these villagers around and weighed their bowel movements. They were passing pounds of shit every day. This kind of diet polishes the lining of the colon, keeping it smooth and exfoliated. And it prevents hemorrhoids and fissures.

He then went to England where people hardly eat vegetables but instead consume loads of processed flour as we do. He weighed their bowel movements, and they were maybe putting out a couple of ounces a day. It's no wonder that colon cancer, which is in part caused by a poor diet, is a major health problem in the developed world.

maintenance

45

Another well-known aid for healthy bowel function is exercise. When you're moving around, your intestines are more active too, encouraging peristalsis (the wavelike action of the instestines that moves the stool along).

So a moist, bulky stool is achieved from water, roughage, and exercise—and not from laxatives. Laxatives are irritants. They incite the colon to push the stool along. But they can become addictive, in that we develop a tolerance and have to take stronger and stronger laxatives to achieve the same results. There are bulk laxatives, which are really just concentrated fiber (e.g. Metamucil). These are not harmful, and if you prefer to take them, go ahead.

Remember, frequency of bowel movements is individual. You don't have to have a bowel movement every day to be healthy. As women, our hormones tend to relax smooth muscles and the colon is a smooth muscle. So we may not be as "regular" as men. If you have no abdominal or rectal discomfort and it's been a day or two since you moved your bowels, relax. If you're uncomfortable, if you feel intestinal spasms, if you feel that there's some big rock there that you can't push out, then you may have a problem and should probably seek professional help. Very, very occasional use (and by this we mean when there's an event, like traveling, moving, or constipation as a corollary to some other medical problem) of laxatives is all right, but the key word here is occasional.

LABIA MAJORA

To recap, the labia majora are the fatty lips of the vagina, which are usually covered in hair. They are filled with a plexus of veins and the mysterious Bartholin's gland. Some people theorize that this gland makes a smell that attracted cavemen. The medical community has no idea what the gland's purpose (if it has one) is today.

The duct that connects the gland to the outside world terminates at the vaginal opening. If that duct gets plugged up with mucus, the material the gland excretes backs up into the labia, causing swelling, and sometimes an infection. If it's not infected, we call it a Bartholin's duct cyst. If it is infected, it's called a Bartholin's duct abscess and needs to be drained. Once or twice, there have been reports of women whose Bartholin's cyst became cancerous, though this is one of the rarest malignancies.

After sex, if you've worn tight pants all day, or whenever you feel that your labia are swollen, a hot bath or warm compress can loosen whatever is plugging up the duct and prevent you from developing a somewhat painful problem. But if you don't catch it early, see your doctor who will reopen your duct with a procedure called *marsupialization*, where the cyst is cut open and sutured to ensure an open channel. Another new procedure is called the Wurm Catheter, which remains inflated inside the plugged duct, keeping it open for at least a week. When it's removed, a permanent channel remains. This approach is more attractive to some, since it is quicker and more easily performed in a doctor's office as opposed to an operating room. On the other hand, you're sitting on a catheter (i.e. a hollow, plastic tube) for a week, which can be uncomfortable. You also have to care for the catheter, taking warm baths ensuring that it doesn't plug up.

PERINEUM

At the opening of the vagina, there's a fold of tissue that's part of the perineum (the area between the rectum and the vagina). This part of the vestibule can be easily traumatized during vaginal intercourse, and many women will get something like a paper cut. As you can imagine, this makes sex very painful. Given time and rest, it will heal, but once the cut is there, it is easily opened again and can become a chronic fissure. Occasionally the fissure refuses to heal and the only treatment is to cut out the aggravated tear and sew fresh tissue together.

If you can prevent this problem from persisting, you will save yourself a whole lot of grief. If you notice that sex is uncomfortable, try to change your angle. If you notice that you are not as well lubricated as you might like, put a lot of goo on the spot that hurts. This goo rule is a guideline that comes in handy for a host of sexually associated vaginal discomforts.

A friend realized late in the game that the woman he had taken to bed was a virgin, and came tearing down the hall one night screaming, "I need lubrication!" So we're looking in the kitchen and the medicine cabinet and all through our rooms to help this guy out. He went back with Brylcream and later claimed it worked "like a dream." Of course, this was a temporary measure. You're better off with natural stuff like olive oil and egg whites if you're desperate than you are with products that contain perfume or alcohol. If you're in a bind, you will find something in your house that will do the job; just use common sense. If you're using a condom (and you most probably should be), avoid oil-based lubricants like Vaseline, which tend to break down latex and may cause the condom to tear.

LABIA MINORA

The labia minora have a lot of sweat glands and nerve endings. After the clitoris, they are the most sensitive part of our genitalia, and after our armpits, they can be the smelliest part of our body. The only potential problems with the labia minora are mechanical ones—e.g. they can get pulled into the vagina by a penis or other foreign body. Sometimes it's necessary to manually move the labia and then insert the penis. The same goes for inserting a diaphragm or a tampax; if you need to, just spread the labia and get them out of the way.

CLITORIS

Like the vagina, the clitoris is covered by a very delicate mucus membrane. If you are going to have any prolonged activity in that area, best to lubricate it. Really, use anything in a pinch. Natural lubrication can be plenty, but if it isn't, don't hesitate to help your body out. Again, though, steer clear of Vaseline and other oil-based lubricants, which can cause a condom to tear.

* * * * *

Bidets

The first time most North Americans travel to Europe, they're mystified by the second toiletlike accoutrement in their bathroom. This is a bidet (biDAY), and it's Europe's solution to the smelly crotch problem. Instead of just wiping their behinds with toilet paper, they get a little soap and water together and use the bidet, which shoots water in an upward stream for direct cleaning action.

MOTHER: "Remember that first trip to France when you were six?"

DAUGHTER: "Like it was yesterday."

MOTHER: "Very funny. Well, half the time we looked for parks and ponies and petting zoos, and the other half we ate."

DAUGHTER: "Sounds about right."

MOTHER: "And my jeans kept getting tighter and tighter, and I wound up taking long hot baths at every hotel in Burgundy."

DAUGHTER: "Because..."

MOTHER: "That's right—Bartholin's cyst because of you."

DAUGHTER: "Thanks, Mom. You're the best."

Aesthetics

I've seen tattoos, labial rings, clitoral rings (ouch!), and I know there are some very personal decorative proclivities out there. As long as these apparati are applied in a sterile environment, there should be no health risk.

chapter five

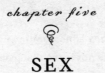

SEX

Into each life a little rain must fall. Almost every woman I know has experienced the unfortunate cliché of sleeping with a guy and never hearing from him again. You review every detail of the event, looking for the reason why why WHY? You examine your physique, your face, your hair, your underwear. You try a different deodorant, a new perfume. You go on a diet. You scour magazines for sex advice columns. You interrogate your friends on their boudoir behavior. But in the end, let me tell you, it had nothing to do with you. Relax. The jerks are out there, and sometimes they fly in under the radar. It even happened to me once, and boy did it make me feel crappy. Thanks a lot, Ian MacGregor, you lobster-touting dickhead.

The best defense you have against the host of STDs is to know your partner. It's embarrassing and it takes balls, but it never hurts to gently request a short medical history from your partner: Has he ever had herpes, gonorrhea, or chlamydia? Has a previous girlfriend ever told him that she caught something from him? Has he been tested for HIV? These are not questions to save for the moment when the penis is at the vaginal opening, because at that point he'll tell you he's Jesus just to get that penis on the road. The days of the anonymous sexual encounter are over. Be smart. Protect your vagina.

We can't say this too many times: maintaining gynecological health requires monogamy. We're not just talking about using condoms, which are absolutely essential, but also a certain amount of care in partner selection. The more people you kiss, the more likely you are to catch a cold. Unfortunately, the things you catch through intercourse are not always curable.

FOREPLAY

Despite everything you've seen in the latest romantic comedy, going from fully clothed to full penetration is not exactly the express bus to a satisfying sexual experience. Most women need to warm up the motor before they take the Ferrari out for a spin. Communicate with your partner. Tell him or her what you personally need to get the most out of your sexual experience.

We can't provide guidelines for what will be the best pre-penetration routine for you. Some women need oral sex, some women hate oral, some women want to touch themselves, some women never touch themselves (even though they should), and there are those women who, despite what we've just said, like to go straight to the main event. We can't tell you how you feel—think of it as a journey of self-discovery.

It's a mantra. Nothing is in any way wrong between or among *consenting adults*. The tantamount thing to remember is that no two people have the exact same sexual responsiveness, desires, or fantasies. Take any three teenage girls and they all have tremendous crushes on three different movie stars. With me, it was Marlon Brando while Guy Madison was IT for my best friend, Patty Giangreco.

* * * * *

MOTHER: "I saw *On The Waterfront* twelve times."

DAUGHTER: "You did?"

MOTHER: "Well, seven times. Not to mention *The Wild One*, *Streetcar Named Desire*, and *The Men*. He was a fabulous paraplegic."

DAUGHTER: "Nice, Mom."

* * * * *

THE DEED

The act of vaginal intercourse, which is a pretty bare bones sexual experience, is a penis going into a vagina, thrusting for (hopefully) a while, and then ejaculating the product of that event into the vagina. That ejaculate is theoretically loaded with sperm. The sperm go to the egg and the woman gets pregnant. It shouldn't be news to you that sex is primarily a form of reproduction. Fortunately, we humans have massive brains, and we quickly learned to take advantage of the fringe benefits of sexual intercourse.

Over the millennia, we've developed the scope of our sexual activities and refined our tastes. It's analogous to food; we used to eat half-rotten mammoth meat and now we like tuna melts and soufflé. Of course, even in the cave, our ancestors probably enjoyed fresh meat a

You Probably Know More than Mom Did

It's not like anyone's born knowing about sex or their bodies or the other sex's bodies. My older cousin Leonard, the doctor, told me about a woman in his anatomy class in medical school. They were working on the male genitalia, and she kept cutting and cutting and cutting, until finally Leonard asked, "What are you looking for?" And she said, "The bone." And Leonard laughed and laughed, and I'm thinking, "There's no bone?"

Sex was in many ways tricky for the average woman in the first half of the twentieth century. When I was growing up in the fifties, many women felt that there was a very fine line between appropriately enjoying sex and appearing to be a nymphomaniac whore. Halfway through the century, there seemed to be a change of mind (or many minds). A college textbook of mine credited the soldiers returning from Europe who had experienced women who seemed to actually like sex. So perhaps they encouraged their girlfriends at home to enjoy what went on in the bedroom. But, who can say? Maybe people in the American bedroom back in the 1950's had heaps of kinky sex—we just don't talk about it like they do over in France.

great deal more than a carcass that had been sitting around for a while. The same is true of sex; it was probably occasionally pleasurable then, but now we have had millennia of improvements that directly and indirectly benefit our sex lives.

You may not actually feel this way. Most people are convinced that everyone is having a better sex life than they are. Lots of people look around and think that all the people around them are masters while they themselves are mere novices. The truth is, we could all get better, and we could all be more communicative. And the other truth is that it just doesn't matter. Whether you're skiing the bunny slope or a black diamond trail, the only thing that matters is that you're enjoying it.

Sex should be fun. We can take ourselves so seriously, at the gym, the doctor's, our friendships, and our sex lives. If you want to try something that doesn't look like you'll break a bone doing it, try it. If you want to try a different position, location, or time of day, make it happen—this keeps variety in your relationship.

When it comes to the nitty-gritty, believe me, I am no sex expert, but I can tell you a thing or two I've picked up. Sex therapists believe the most therapeutic position is with the woman on top, because there's no sense of being overwhelmed. The woman maintains control, so she can angle herself so the penis enters the vagina in the direction that best suits her. And of course, the clitoris is accessible for a little extravaginal stimulation. For a woman that feels uncomfortable or a sense of being smothered when she's on the bottom, it's worthwhile to give this a try. That's not to say that being on top will be your favorite position ultimately, but it's a good jumping-off point for a woman who's trying to figure out her own body.

ORAL SEX

Ah, oral sex. Nowhere in the lexicon of female sexual activity do opinions skew so greatly. We'd say most women hope and pray for oral sex, but there's a sizeable minority for whom it's uncomfortably intimate and a smaller minority who will not tolerate it. In many cases, discomfort with oral sex is a direct corollary to insecurity and ignorance about one's vagina. If you don't like your crotch because it's smelly and messy, you're not going to let your boyfriend put his face in it.

For those of you who are interested in oral sex, just remember to communicate effectively. You wouldn't believe how confusing the vagina and its environs can be to men—many are pretty much lost

---

Our Rules
....
The basic guidelines for sex are pretty intuitive. The first and last rule is to do no harm. Some people associate pain with sex, but I don't think this pain should leave scars or draw blood. Some women like to get slapped around or get a little spanking. Sure, go for it! But if your idea of good sex requires surgical correction, you are in a bad place. And if whatever activity you're engaging in is followed by profuse bleeding, seek medical attention.
....

Other dangers of anal sex include misplaced foreign bodies. Every doctor knows a story about someone who showed up at the emergency room with something stuck in the wrong place. The scariest of these that I've seen was a light bulb in some poor man's rectum, which is an extraordinarily unkind thing to do to another person. They ultimately used obstetrical forceps to remove the light bulb intact, while the patient remained under general anesthesia. A colleague of mine found a jar of Hellman's mayonnaise in a patient's vagina. The lesson here is not to get too wasted and naked with someone you just met. It'll seem like a riot at the time, but you'll be absolutely mortified and probably uncomfortable when you have to go to the hospital.

down there. Speak, point, move, moan, draw a picture, whatever you can do to help out an eager partner is going to dramatically improve both your sex lives.

In general, you're looking for your partner to address your clitoris with his fingers, lips, and tongue. Gently, at first, and then with increasing pressure, he'll probably want to manipulate your clitoris in some fashion that will be unique to you. Circles, back and forth, tapping, sucking, and a hundred other methods we couldn't think of are all worth exploring.

ANAL SEX

Unlike the vagina, the anus is a lens opening. It can widen to a point, which shouldn't be exceeded too terribly much or you risk injury. The key to anal sex, even more so than vaginal sex, is lubrication because there's not really any mechanism back there for smoothing your path. A slow, gentle, greased entry is essential.

The most common health implication for an anal sex aficionada is bringing bacteria from the rectum and introducing it into your vagina, which could cause a raging, nasty infection. If you are going to put a penis or instrument in your butt, that penis or instrument needs to be *thoroughly* cleaned before it meets up with your vagina again.

ORGASMS

An orgasm is physically manifested by a neuragenic (i.e. starting in your nerves) release simultaneously throughout the body, coupled with involuntary contractions of the vagina. And it feels great. Orgasms for women are not essential for reproduction, so not a whole lot of scientific effort has been directed this way. Also, decades ago, it probably seemed a little dangerous to encourage women to have orgasms, because if sex was that great for her, maybe she'd look for it outside of the marriage bed.

According to Masters and Johnson, the first stage of sexual excitement involves an increase in pulse, respiration, perspiration, a flush across the chest, increase in vaginal lubrication, and a swelling or engorgement of the walls of the vagina, labia, and clitoris. This concert of events is hopefully followed by the orgasm, which can be described as involuntary contractions of the entire reproductive tract, and an overwhelming wave of pleasure and release, followed by a sense of well-being and sleepiness. We'd like to give you something more personal, but we had to draw the line somewhere.

WHERE'S MY ORGASM?

If you don't have orgasms, well, that's something to think about. The word frigidity is no longer used in medicine. This was the term coined in the thirties for women who were not orgasmic. Not only was it inappropriate, it was judgmental. The term we use now is preorgasmic, meaning that you just haven't had your orgasm yet. Approximately 11 percent of women in this country fall into this category.

Lack of orgasm is caused by a physical problem less than 1 percent of the time. Physical causes for being orgasmically challenged

I had a patient who was eighty-two and told me that she was preorgasmic. I said, "Good for you!" She was seeing a sex therapist. Better late than never. I hope she lives long enough.

usually involve being on certain medications (like Prozac). Structural problems that would lead to this sad outcome are fortunately very rare. There are, however, an infinite number of nonphysical reasons for preorgasmia that account for the overwhelming majority of cases.

Even though they are rare, the first thing I do for preorgasmic women is eliminate physical problems. Does it hurt when you have sex? No one is going to have an orgasm if they're in pain (unless that's your "thing"). Inadequate lubrication is the number one problem. Some women have a vaginal infections that disrupt their pleasure. Some women have endometriosis so it can be painful when a penis goes in the wrong direction. Some women are so tense and fearful that they cannot relax and allow penetration without pain, and if they can't relax enough for penetration, an orgasm is going to be really tough.

The second thing I do is give them a mirror and show them their anatomy. Even some patients with very helpful, loving, eager boyfriends have said, "Oh. THAT'S where the clitoris is!" Sometimes just showing them where things are leads to pleasurable results.

GET OFF!

Masturbation is very important for the preorgasmic woman (okay, for all women). It's impossible to tell another person what gives you pleasure if you can't give yourself pleasure. Think about how difficult it would be to show someone how to play the piano if you'd never seen one before. Take a mirror and look. Touch, and figure out what feels good or feels not so good to you.

The Clitoris Ain't Perfect

Women have inquired about surgery to move the clitoris closer to the vagina. This is probably a bad idea, in that moving it would cut off its nerve supply. Another flimsy theory on improving women's sexual responsiveness is to "unhood" the clitoris (removing the fold that covers it). This is fraught with risk. The clitoris is so sensitive that it's a short hop from pleasure to pain. These women may have trouble sitting down or wearing tight pants, and forget about horseback riding. This is not an operation that has ever been popular. Conversely, a hundred years ago, removing the clitoris was not uncommon in New York City for women who were "too demanding." Thanks again, J. Marion Sims. (See page 34 for more on this major figure of gynecology.)

There are all kinds of masturbatory techniques that have been written about extensively. We don't know them all, because you stick with what works best for you. Some women masturbate on their stomachs, some on their backs, some in the shower, some in the bath, some with their fingers, some with the palms of their hands, and some with their vibrators. A technique that's promoted for beginners involves water—a handheld shower massager will work, or if you're limber enough to get yourself underneath the bathtub faucet, put your legs up

Camaraderie in Masturbation

I was at a spa that included a huge, twenty-person hot tub in the women's locker room. As I climbed in, a woman was getting out, looking very relaxed. She said to me, "Third spigot on the left." I was only there for a weekend, and every time I checked, that spigot was occupied. Finally, on Sunday afternoon, that special spigot was available, and she was absolutely right. It was wonderful.

From a gynecological perspective, Sigmund Freud was a total asshole. His ideas about life and women were pretty ridiculous; he believed that a vaginal orgasm was the goal and that somehow this was the only real orgasm. He felt that if you had to directly stimulate the clitoris, then the orgasm was inferior or childlike, and don't get us started on all that "penis envy." This stuff is total bullshit. Any orgasm you have, clitoral, vaginal or other, is just fantastic.

on either side and let it rip. You can just lie there with the water running over your clitoris, and if you wait long enough, most women will reach a peak.

Once you've had an orgasm, you can usually reproduce it. The trick is getting that first one. You have to coordinate a huge number of variables in order to find your way to a place that you haven't been to before. You should almost definitely focus on the clitoris as a starting point. For 99.99 percent of women, an orgasm involves direct or indirect stimulation to the clitoris. We don't want to discount anyone's particular experience, but for most women out there, the vaginal orgasm will forever be a nagging illusion. Of course, there are all kinds of stories about the rare woman who had her clitoris removed but can still have orgasms. There are transsexuals who don't have clitorides and have orgasms with a synthetic, surgically constructed vagina. I certainly can't explain every orgasm.

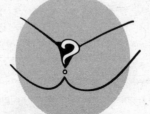

Orgasms are wonderful, but they don't keep you healthy. You won't die if you don't have one. There are women who say they've tried everything. They enjoy sex, they get excited, but they just don't have orgasms. Maybe working with a sex therapist would help, but if they're happy, then that's the most important thing.

On the other hand, I had a patient who said she was really, really busy; she was married to a really, really busy man; and together they had really, really busy lives so they didn't have that much time for sex. I said, "What frequency are we talking about here?" and she told me that they were having intercourse maybe once a year. I suggested to her that this might be a red flag. She said, "I'm happy. My husband's happy." If two people are truly comfortable with their sex lives, no matter how meager it may seem, who am I to say there's something wrong?

But the time came when they wanted kids, and this really, really busy couple was having sex maybe twice a year. And I said, "Well, you're really not gonna get lucky with twice a year, so maybe we should consider sex therapy." It turned their lives around.

The couple went for therapy and developed a love for sex. They realized they'd had major communication problems. She got pregnant within several months, and they continued their sex therapy through-

He Came, She Came

A guy who can withhold his orgasm is considered a great lover. A woman who takes too long is a drag. Why are we expected to have orgasms at the drop of a hat and a man is heroic if he can hold out? Nobody has quick orgasms all the time. You're stressed at work, you're overtired, you've got a slight headache, you're stiff from going to the gym, whatever the cause, it may take you a while to warm up. Other times, you've been thinking about it all day, you can't wait to get home, you're excited before you open the front door, and BOOM.

out the pregnancy. She told me she was the only client wearing maternity clothes in the waiting room at the sex therapist's office.

I don't mean to sound fanatical about sex, but, in my opinion, the improvement in her sex life changed this woman's whole life. Beforehand, she was rather obnoxious, and afterwards, she became a very affable, cheerful woman with two kids, a husband who adored her, and a great sex outlook. And there was a really simple solution.

But not everyone gets miracles. Orgasms can rock your world, but it doesn't hurt to be realistic. One young patient asked if she could be having orgasms and not know it. The sex therapist I called said it had been known to happen that a woman could have such high expectations that they missed the real deal while they were waiting for the earth to move. I've also had older patients say, "You know, I used to be able to do it four times a day, and my orgasms used to be violent. Now, I'm sixty and my orgasms are okay, but...."

TEENAGERS AND SEX

TEENAGERS ARE HAVING SEX?!?!?!

Teenage girls are having sex. Not all of them, certainly, and maybe not even most of them. But a lot of them. And they're all thinking about it. This is not a manifesto; this is biology. At puberty, for girls and boys alike, there's a natural urge to investigate these strange and wonderful feelings. It is the height of stupidity to say, "let's just tell them to say 'no.'" According to Columbia University and the *New York Times*, the majority of teens who pledge abstinence have sex anyway, and most of those who do fail to protect themselves against STDs.*

Each girl matures at her own pace. And some may be ready for sexual experiences sooner than others, or sooner than you might think, or sooner than you may like. On the other hand, it's a very sad thing when girls have sex for the wrong reasons. Peer pressure and a tremen-

@vaginas

* Jane Brody, "Abstinence Only—Does it Work?" *The New York Times* , June 1, 2004.

... was the title of a book in our parochial school library that only sen-
iors were allowed to read. At eighteen, most of the girls were about to
get married. This book was touted as a helpful introduction to sex in
marriage even though it didn't say one useful thing. On the plus side,
sex was presented as nothing to be afraid of. On the other hand, it was
made clear that sex was a wifely duty and was therefore a sin to refuse.
So it was a sin to say "no" to your husband, but also a sin to say "yes"
to anyone else. I know they meant well, but nuns really aren't qualified
to teach sex education.

dous desire to be popular or in the "in" crowd are all terribly real and
important to adolescents.

THE LOWDOWN ON HYMENS

The hymen is a membrane at the vaginal opening, approximately an
inch inside your body, at the beginning of the vagina. There are all different sorts of hymens. Some are thick and inhospitable to visitors
while others are barely there and broach no barrier to a vaginal guest.
The vast majority of hymens don't deter tampons, but you may bleed
when you first have sex as he/she stretches the hymen. Very rarely,
there are women whose hymens seem impermeable. Hymenotomies,
minor surgery that broadens the hymen, are extremely rare. These are
also performed on the few women who have too small an opening to
release their menstrual blood. Regardless of what happens to the mysti-
cal hymen, you are a virgin until you are sexually active

MOM'S ADVICE FOR THE PARENTS

Unconditional love is absolutely essential. Nothing that happens will
ever compromise your love for your child forever and ever to the maximum. If your child doesn't wish to tell you something, if she's being
discreet, or if there are things she doesn't want to share with you, that's

one thing. But if she is afraid to tell you something that she actually *needs* to tell you, then you have lost.

Boredom is your enemy. A bored teenager will do things she would never think of doing if she were busy, active, engaged in extracurricular activities, vacations, family get-togethers, etc. I believe that the best thing for a rambunctious teenager is physical activity. Any activity is distracting, but physical activity is not only healthy, it provides stress relief. Sports are a great way for teenagers to spend all that surplus energy that might otherwise be used elsewhere.

If you talk to your teenage daughter only *once* about sex, urge/beg/plead with her to use condoms. Talking about sex is not issuing your daughter a license to have sex; just as sweeping it under the carpet will not make it go away. Also, offering to take her to a gynecologist if she would feel more comfortable talking to a professional is very appropriate. Buying her a book like this one is another good idea.

LIZ'S ADVICE FOR THE GIRLS

The only person who really knows if you're ready to have sex with another person is you. However, just because you're sure you're ready, doesn't mean that your partner is, that the situation is right, that he or she is the right person, etc. etc. etc.

If you feel any pressure in the situation, then remove yourself from it. Ultimately, I promise you, no one is going to like you less if you aren't sexually active. One of the most important lessons I've learned is that people will actually like you more if you can think for yourself and stand by what you personally believe, *especially* when you distinguish yourself from the crowd.

As for a guy who threatens to break up with you if you won't sleep with him, he's unequivocally not worth your time. Believe me, I know these guys now, and in their midtwenties, they've become a collection of balding, tubby, assholes who puzzle over why they can't get laid.

You're going to remember the experience for the rest of your life. The most important elements are mutual respect, comfort with one another, and enough emotional maturity to handle *all* the possible repercussions of the act. I know it doesn't sound that romantic, but it is the truth.

Even less romantic is the oftentimes reality of the situation, which is awkward, sometimes uncomfortable, disorienting, etc. Being a virgin means being a novice, a first-timer, a beginner. You can't expect to jump on your first pair of skis and be an Olympic gold medallist. Like all things, it takes patience and practice. Unlike most things, practicing is a lot of fun.

INFERTILITY AND SEX

The saddest sexual problem is when people get wrapped up in fertility, and all of a sudden, they're having sex by the clock, at different frequencies, around ovulation, and men are masturbating in the doctor's bathroom with a magazine. This can really injure a sexual relationship. It's called "work fucking." It's pitiful. These people break my heart.

When a couple is hell-bent on conception, it's not uncommon for the man to develop sexual problems, i.e. erectile dysfunction. For a man, to be told he has to perform at a given time because his wife is ovulating and she's waiting to be inseminated must be the worst, unsexiest sensation. Meanwhile, the woman is taking her temperature and doing her ovulation predictor kit, taking her fertility drugs, and I'm telling them what the best time and frequency is for them to have sex. It's very hard to maintain a "this is fun" attitude. You both start to feel like, "We have to have sex again. I was hoping I could watch the baseball game."

One thing to remember is that because you have to have sex at certain times doesn't mean you can't have sex the rest of the month just for fun. When you're horny, please have sex. Try to remember what it was like when you were doing it just for fun. Try to avoid morphing lovemaking into a baby-making operation.

If you are under thirty, I urge you to remember that a year of trying to get pregnant could be a year of great sex. Don't look at the clock. Don't think about the eggs. Just try to think of a new place to have sex.

The first month your father and I were going to try and get pregnant, I figured out the weekend I was going to be ovulating. I said, "Let's go away somewhere romantic, with a fireplace, a four-poster bed, down quilts, fluffy pillows, potpourri, and candles." I found a hotel that sounded charming, but when we got there, it was loaded with kids. It was like a motel at Disney Land, and how unsexy is that? It rained non-stop, fostering this disgusting musty smell in our room. So we had sex, and then I said, "Okay, we have to wait thirty-six hours for your sperm to reaccumulate." Your father said, "You mean we can't do it for fun anymore? But it's raining out." I told him to read a book.

By Saturday, the motel had become unbearable. So we went somewhere else where it was also raining, miserable, and cold. I launched into a series of crying jags because I'd decided I was definitely infertile. Finally we found an inn that could offer us a room with a fireplace, but what happens when you try to light a fire with wet wood? It took about forty-five seconds for the room to fill with smoke. Meanwhile, we were on a set of twin cots, which kept sliding apart and depositing us on the floor. After three minutes, we were coughing so much from the smoke, we had to leave the room anyway. All I ended up with was a really bad cold, and I didn't get pregnant.

Brainstorm about a new sexy outfit. Find a new food to play with in bed (or on the kitchen counter). Because you will look back with regret if you make this unpleasant. Enjoy yourself. If you are over thirty, the rules may change slightly, and if you are over forty, they absolutely change because by then, time has become your enemy.

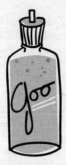

MISCELLANEOUS SEX ISSUES

Some fortunate people have a lot of sex, especially in the early passionate beginnings of a relationship. That's really not what the vagina is designed for. Inside, it's all thin mucus membranes, which are very delicate. We're not saying, "Don't have too much sex," but rather, "Be sensitive to your body's needs." Use plenty of goo.

A whole lot of sex can also heat up the walls of your vagina, causing the fungus that naturally lives there to grow out of control and into a yeast infection. The thrusting penis can push bacteria up into the bladder, causing an infection. We call this particular problem "honey-

Bigger and Brawnier Isn't Always Better

Vaginal trauma is very common with what's called "rough sex." I did a rotation in Jamaica in the West Indies where apparently very forceful thrusting is the style. Women would come to the emergency room almost every night with lacerations at the top of the vagina and at the vaginal opening. Size can also be a factor. I would say maybe fewer than six times in my career has a patient complained that her husband's penis was too small, but dozens of women have complained about a sexual partner's penis being too big. Size can require excessive lubrication, a slow gentle, entry and a careful negotiation of position. Size plus style can be very traumatic.

moon cystitis" because it's almost always caused by a precipitous upswing in sexual activity. This is not uncommon—women have "commuter" relationships and are only able to see boyfriends or partners on weekends. They squeeze all their sex into a weekend and on Monday, the woman has a burning sensation when she urinates.

Remember to drink a lot of water and urinate after intercourse (flushing out the bladder). After three goes, everything gets a little tired. Even when the mind is willing, the body can struggle. We've said it before and we're saying it again—goo is the answer. KY Jelly is the obvious choice, but there's sure to be something in your house that will work in a pinch: egg whites, saliva, and olive oil are all good last minute options.

* * * * *

DAUGHTER: "That was sweet."

MOTHER: "What?"

DAUGHTER: "Not the story about Jamaica, but you know, earlier... That stuff about keeping the lines of communication open and being nonjudgmental about when I was a teenager and sex and everything..."

MOTHER: "You've had sex?"

chapter six

CONTRACEPTION

There was a time not so long ago when people risked their lives and freedom to deliver reproductive choice to the women of this country. We're very fortunate to be the beneficiaries of their pioneering efforts, as it seems there are now unlimited options for avoiding unwanted pregnancies. There are contraceptive methods for women of all habits; be you lazy, forgetful, meticulous, controlling, or medication averse.

Sadly, there are far fewer options for protecting yourself against diseases and infections. It may not be your first pick overall, but when you initiate a new sexual relationship, you only have one choice, which is really no choice at all—condoms.

Through recorded history back to the ancient tablets of the Assyrians, the two universal medical preoccupations have been contraception and pain relief in childbirth. Many medical breakthroughs have stemmed from both. As far as contraception, we've come a long way from infanticide, which was standard in some cultures for imperfect or unwanted babies. Most advances in contraception have evolved in the last hundred years or so, which parallels the rise of women's rights. This is no coincidence. We're not at the mercy of our reproductive organs anymore.

Manifesto stated, the fact remains that whenever a penis goes in a vagina, pregnancy is a possibility. Of course, women don't get pregnant every time they have sexual intercourse, but you never know when or where it might happen.

The youngest pregnancy on record was a girl named Linda Medina. She was from South America and five when she conceived. Linda's father was also the father of her baby. Precocious (early) puberty, a rare disorder, revealed his crime.

There is no absolute protection against unwanted pregnancy short of celibacy. Every contraceptive method has established pregnancy rates both for "perfect use" (a theoretical number that conjectures how effective a particular method is if used exactly right) and "regular use" (how we imperfect humans actually follow instructions). So while you can never have intercourse with the guarantee that you won't get pregnant, for most, it's worth the small risk. Life without sex would be so dull!

SYSTEMIC HORMONAL TREATMENTS

Of all your options, systemic hormonal treatments offer the most flexible, and effective protection against pregnancy as well as a host of corollary health benefits. Within this category, there are several options that vary in content (which hormones) and method of delivery (how they are introduced into your body). Systemic contraceptives either contain estrogen and progesterone or just progesterone, and the delivery methods include pills, shots, patches, rings, and IUDs (intrauterine devices). The premier form of systemic contraception, and still the most popular by a vast margin, is the life-changing, history-making birth control pill.

THE LIFE-CHANGING, HISTORY-MAKING
BIRTH CONTROL PILL

A Brief History of the Pill

The pill was developed in the fifties based on the premise that the menstrual cycle can be modified so that there is no follicle of the month, and therefore, no egg released when a woman is given estrogen and/or progesterone in any combination. Remember, the pituitary stimulates the ovary to make estrogen and progesterone. Then these hormones travel back through the bloodstream, past the pituitary. Seeing these hormones, the pituitary says, "Aha, I've stimulated the ovary. My work is done here." Therefore it doesn't make its other hormones—FSH and LH—that stimulate the ovary to produce a ripe follicle. No follicle = no egg. No egg = no baby. You only menstruate when you stop taking the pill, cease the hormonal flow, and your body thinks it's time to shed the lining of the uterus and restart your cycle.

* * * * *

DAUGHTER: "So, Mom, if you're on the pill your whole life, do you have lots of eggs left over when you go off. Like could you just stay on the pill and then have all your kids when you're sixty?"

MOTHER: "Nope. Nobody knows why you don't have eggs left if you're on the pill you're whole life. There's more to this than we know—more hormones in the brain, more hormones being made by the ovary, and some internal clock that says, 'Time for menopause.' If you have a million eggs left, and the clock says it's time, you'll use them all within the time allotted."

* * * * *

When the pill was first developed, they didn't know quite what was going to happen. Chemists suggested prescribing hormones the way the ovary would, with a one-week cessation period so that the endometrium could shed. They designed this process to mimic a normal cycle of twenty-eight days because physicians were aiming to simulate natural events. Additionally, this synthetic menstrual period was a built-in reassurance that those on the pill weren't pregnant—a valuable piece of information for those first guinea pigs who weren't sure they could trust those little pills.

The first brand of birth control pills was called Enovid. At five milligrams of estrogen per pill, Enovid delivered a relatively huge amount of hormones. Today, pills tend to contain about thirty-five micrograms, or one-third of a milligram. Of course Enovid worked with immediate benefits. Periods were much less painful, if not completely painless for women on the pill, and the uterine lining was much thinner so they enjoyed far less bleeding.

Due to the extraordinarily high amounts of estrogen, however, there were some less appealing side effects. Women on Enovid were a little bloated—like they'd swallowed thirty tons of air. Their breasts were swollen and painful. Despite having what were the symptoms of estrogen overdose, practically none of them wanted to stop taking the pill. There is nothing more gloriously liberating than a woman who can control her reproduction—particularly when it was previously unheard of.

It was not unheard of for women on Enovid to downplay their symptoms in a bid to keep those all-important birth control pills coming, which probably contributed to a few significant problems. These were the days of phlebitis (inflammation of a vein in the calf), blood clots, strokes, and all kinds of vascular changes due to the massive doses of hormones.

The medical community continues to improve on the pill. It seems the hormonal load is as low as possible. At twenty micrograms of estrogen, there was a small increase in pregnancies. So we've probably

At first, the pill engendered a certain measure of fear. What if the ovaries never "woke up" again causing permanent sterility? In the first ten years that the pill was around, doctors made their patients go off oral contraceptives one month each year, just to see that these women got their periods back. Of course, that was the month everybody got pregnant. It seems the ovaries don't notice the difference between three months, three years, or thirty years; whenever you go off the pill, your ovaries spark back to life. There are some rare exceptions when women take several months to start menstruating again called "post-pill suppression." This condition is temporary and uncommon.

bottomed out at thirty, but you never know. Pharmaceutical companies continue to mine the possibilities of the birth control pill. Can it be more convenient? Can it help in other areas of a woman's life? Stay tuned.

The Pill Today

There are two major subsets of pills—monophasic and triphaisal. Monophasic ("one phase") pills are all the same, except for the placebo pills you take at the end of the cycle when you get your period. With triphaisal pills ("three phase"), the hormone dosage changes from week to week. Sometimes the estrogen stays the same and the progesterone changes, sometimes it's vice versa. With some, the hormones increase until just before your period, and with others, the hormones peak in the middle. The advantage to the triphaisic pill is that your overall consumption of hormones at the end of the year is slightly lower, which is making this choice increasingly popular. Also, there is a slight decrease in breakthrough bleeding (see page 74) with triphaisal dosages.

Regardless of which pill you choose, most women will take three weeks of "active" pills followed by one week of placebo pills.

contraception

73

The active pills have hormones in them, while the placebo pills are nothing at all—placeholders in your daily pill schedule. The placebo week is when you get your period, as your body withdraws from its controlled, steady hormone supply.

All birth control pills carry the same set of terrific, important benefits and a small risk. The pill reduces the risk of ovarian cancer; your ovary doesn't function, so cells divide less, meaning fewer cells mutate, which leads to less cancer. The pill reduces endometrial cancer because the lining of your uterus remains thinner than it otherwise would. The pill reduces any condition associated with ovulation, like severe menstrual cramps, anemia due to heavy periods, and even the dreaded and multifaceted PMS. Instead of natural but unpredictable fluctuations, the pill maintains a nice, prescribed hormone level. The pill reduces endometriosis, which needs normal menstruation to perpetuate itself. It reduces pelvic infection, because there's less congestion in your system during your period, so there's less food for bacteria.

Pill Problems

The most common and annoying side effect of the pill is breakthrough bleeding, which is abnormal spotting, or bleeding at the wrong time. We call it *breakthrough* because it happens when the patient escapes the control of the pill. This happens most frequently when you forget a pill and happens very frequently when you start the pill. This is not in any way a medical problem, but the only way to address it while staying on oral contraception is through trial and error. Often you just need a different pill or a different delivery method, and it can be time consuming to find the best personal option.

There is one gynecological condition that is not statistically reduced by the birth control pill—cervical cancer. This particular cancer is caused by the human papilloma virus (HPV—see page 234). Should you contract HPV, there is a chance of developing cervical cancer where there once was none because HPV is the necessary precursor to cervical cancer (this is not to say everyone who gets HPV gets cervical cancer, but that every woman who has cervical cancer had HPV

Remember, the birth control pill does not protect you against any STDs. There is no barrier between you and infection when you're on the pill. Although you may hate it, if you are initiating a new relationship, you still have to use condoms.

first—see page 234). In the U.S., where Pap smears are prevalent, the odds of developing cervical cancer remain extremely low. Unfortunately, women on the pill tend to be more sexually active and less careful about insisting on condoms, thereby exposing themselves to more STDs, including HPV. So this statistic is explained by the unnecessary reality that more women on the pill catch HPV, and therefore more women on the pill are likely to get cervical cancer.

So many people these days have HPV, however, that the correlation between women on the pill and cervical cancer may wane with time. The most current thinking on HPV, sure to be dated even by the time you read this, is that almost every young, sexually active American has this virus or has had this virus at some point. It's usually asymptomatic and seems to leave the system within three to five years.

Blood clots are another source of concern, but only for smokers. Up until thirty-five, there is no significantly increased risk of blood clots, stroke, high blood pressure, heart disease, etc. when you combine smoking and the pill. But as a woman gets older, the significant health risk of smoking plus the minimal risk of the pill equals more than the sum of the two. You may be as much as ten times more likely to have a stroke if you are over thirty-five, smoke, and take the pill. If you fall into this category, look out for chest pain, chronic coughing, and most especially, coughing that produces blood.

* * * * *

contraception

75

DAUGHTER: "But, Mom, why'd I have to go off the pill for my knee surgery?"

MOTHER: "Many rules change when you go in for elective surgery because there is time to foster the optimal preoperative situation. I encourage my patients to be in the best possible shape, eat a high iron diet, and get plenty of sleep. This helps to build immunity and is generally a healthy way to be. Additionally, I insist that patients give up the pill temporarily. The risk of bleeding mishaps—miniscule as it is—is worth avoiding."

* * * * *

In addition to these very real concerns, there are a host of other pill-related issues that are far too numerous to list here. For every one million women on the birth control pill, there are one million unique experiences with or opinions about it. Common complaints include a change in libido, vaginal dryness, bad moods, and bloating. Some people complain of depression while others claim to be much happier. Some women's breasts hurt, while other women's breasts get bigger and they're thrilled. Some women get nauseous, others get hungry. We can attribute plenty of this disparity of experience to an individual's body reacting in its own way to a given condition. Some of it can also be chalked up to the placebo affect and the power of suggestion.

Complaints about the pill tend to be very subjective. For 90 percent of women, there are no symptoms or at least no symptoms that they want to talk to a medical professional about. Ten percent of women on the pill will complain to their doctor about side effects. At least 50 percent of these women's issues are addressed by changing the

@vaginas

dose or delivery method. The remaining 50 percent of the women who complained in the first place feel that their symptoms are unacceptable and discontinue using systemic contraception.

THE PATCH

The patch is a one-and-a-half-inch square, beige sticker hormonal delivery device. Instead of taking a pill every day for twenty-one days, circulating estrogen and progesterone via the stomach lining, the patch transmits the exact same hormones through the skin. It's monophaisic as it's the same patch reapplied each week for three weeks. In the patch-less week, there are no hormones supporting the lining of the uterus, hence menstruation.

The patch is a nice idea if you struggle to remember the pill every day but could probably handle remembering something once each week. For people who have specific liver problems (and should avoid pills that are metabolized through the liver, as the birth control pill is) or trouble swallowing pills, the patch is a good option. Some women with sensitive skin report rashes and irritation under their patch. Athletes or vigorously clean people find the patches fall off after their third game of tennis or their fifth bath in a day. And obese women (over 200 pounds) often cannot use the patch because a less effective hormone dose makes it into the bloodstream.

contraception

77

THE RING

If you can't remember the pill and you are an avid swimmer (for example), the ring might be for you. It's a small, transparent, flexible ring between two and three inches in diameter. You insert it way up to the top of the vagina and leave it there for three weeks. It doesn't obstruct sex and releases the same exact hormones as monophasic pills and the patch. If you're squeamish about sticking your finger up your vagina (even though you shouldn't be), it's probably not for you.

LUNELLE

The once-per-month estrogen and progesterone combined shot, Lunelle, should be returning to the American market in the near future. When first released, the dosage was too low and there was an uptick in pregnancy rates. They're working on equivocating the dose of the shot (given once every thirty days) to the dose of the pill (taken each day). It's unclear if Lunelle will require a monthly doctor's visit or if self-injection will be an option. The only opportunity for error is in remembering the shot each month. The drawback is that once you get the injection, you have to ride out the hormones for the full month even if they cause adverse affects. With the pill, you can stop taking it and it's out of your system within a few days.

PROGESTERONE

The mechanical difference between taking the standard estrogen plus progesterone systemic contraception and progesterone alone is that with progesterone alone, you still ovulate each month, but the uterus remains an untenable place for a fertilized egg. It works like this: you're on progesterone alone and you have sex. Your body may have released an egg that month, and the sperm may in fact fertilize that egg. But progesterone makes the lining of the uterus inhospitable, and it is impossible for the fertilized egg to find a home in there. Additionally, progesterone alters the mucus in your vagina (see page 18).

Progesterone pills are predominately for women who can't or won't take estrogen but want the same benefits of the conventional

Remember Norplant, the long-lasting progesterone delivery system? You may recall seeing advertisements for the small, plastic rods inserted under the skin of the upper arm. Those little sticks released progesterone in a continuous fashion for up to seven years. Problems arose when it came time to remove the device: and often scars had formed around the sticks and they had to be surgically removed. So they're back to the drawing board with Norplant.

estrogen and progesterone pill. This works well for women who are breast-feeding and cannot take estrogen because it suppresses lactation. Other ailments that lead women to this particular choice include certain vascular problems that cause blood clots. These women are often advised to stay away from estrogen. If you fall into either category and are attached to your birth control pills, discuss the progesterone-only options with your doctor.

PROGESTERONE SHOTS

Depo Provera is the brand name for the progesterone shot administered every three months. The upside is that you only have to remember to get your shot every three months and it's extremely effective. Additionally, this method ultimately causes the lining of the uterus to be so thin, you don't get a period at all. For these reasons, it's very popular with younger women.

THE MORNING AFTER PILL IS JUST THE SAME OLD PILL

So you're having this fabulous sexual experience with someone you just started dating. You've already gotten past the uncomfortable bit and he's happily wearing a condom. But then it breaks. You quickly do the math. . . . It's day fourteen, and you're ovulating! Millions of sperm are swimming as hard as their little tails can propel them towards that inno-

contraception

79

cent little egg. You know that it takes a couple of days for all those eager sperm to get up to the egg, where they may succeed in fertilizing it. Four days later, it will be ready to implant in the uterus.

Somebody brilliant said, "Wait a minute! Progesterone alters the lining of the uterus and makes it inhospitable to a fertilized egg. Let's administer a lot of hormones right now." When the fertilized egg shows up, it can't find a home. It swims around looking for a good spot, and when it can't find one, it dies.

This is how the "morning after pill" or emergency contraception works, and it's very simple. Take four or five (depending on the brand) active birth control pills immediately after the worrisome encounter. Twelve hours later, take four or five more. If there's any question of your being asleep or forgetting the second dose of four pills, take all eight at once. To be precise, ask your gynecologist exactly how many of the particular brand of pill you should take to prevent pregnancy after unprotected sex, as with some stronger pills, you can effectively take fewer.

It's nearly impossible to conjecture how effective this method is, because we have little way of knowing how many women who take it would have gotten pregnant if they hadn't. Depending on where you are in your cycle, the chances can be as high as 25 percent that you'll get pregnant during unprotected intercourse. You probably reduce that risk by 75 percent with the morning after pill.

There are two companies that package the morning after pill in its own little kit; one's called Preven and the other is Plan B. Plan B is progesterone only, while Preven is the traditional estrogen and progesterone birth control pills. In an unprecedented political maneuver, the head of the FDA recently vetoed Plan B's application to be sold over the counter. However, if there's no twenty-four-hour drug store in your neighborhood, any girlfriend on the pill can rush over with a package of pills right away. If that's not doable, don't hesitate to call your gynecologist. I AM THRILLED to prescribe this to help save a patient from misery and heartache. Remember though, after the morning after pill, you need to have an STD screen at your next doctor's appointment (see page 84).

Am I going to gain weight?
(This is the *most* frequently asked question)
Once sensational misinformation has gained a popular foothold, it's almost impossible to eradicate it. One of the most common of these myths is that you're going to gain weight on the pill. Blind studies have scientifically concluded that weight gain is not a side effect of the birth control pill. Ninety-five to ninety-eight percent of women on the pill have no problem with this whatsoever. Some women lose weight. Some women gain weight. They all blame the pill.

There is probably some validity to the argument that if you believe that you will gain weight, then you will. There are also behavioral differences that may go unnoticed. For example, when you first go on the pill, it's easy to pin any coincidental weight gain on those innocent pink tablets. Some new-to-the-pill patients have told me that they start saying things like, "I might as well have another piece of cake; I'm on the pill."

What if I miss a day? Should I take two immediately?
Every day you miss your pill, you're adding another half a percentage point of pregnancy risk, because you've allowed the ovary to wake up a little bit. Missing a pill increases the risk that you'll start shedding the lining of the uterus, so you may have some bleeding. Traditionally, we have told patients to double up on the pill the next day, which may help. Now, I usually tell my patients to continue with one pill each day until the package is finished, because it's less disruptive. This method costs you a fraction of 1 percent in terms of pregnancy avoidance, so if you're not too sensitive to your pill and want to be extra safe, go ahead and take two to make up for the one you missed.

What if I miss more than one day?
You must use alternate methods of contraception if you've missed two days of your birth control pill. The safest way to proceed is to cease

contraception

81

taking the pill for seven days, start a new pack on the eighth day, and you'll be protected again after another seven days—so you're inconvenienced for two weeks.

If you really need to have sex without a condom for some reason, and you're at the last week of your pack (i.e. you're going to get your period the next week), you can trick your body into only a week's worth of inconvenience. Toss the incomplete pack, and begin a fresh one with no risk of pregnancy. If you skipped two pills in the first two weeks of your package, it's much more likely to result in inadvertent ovulation. Toss the pack, start again in seven days, and you're okay seven days after that.

No matter how you handle it, if you're missing pills all the time, you are at risk for an unwanted pregnancy, and may want to consider the patch, ring, or shot.

Are there any future fertility risks?

The pill improves your fertility because if your ovaries are quiet, they and, by extension, you are more likely to stay healthy. In circumventing your body's natural hormonal cycle, the pill suppresses cell activity and division, lessening the chances of cell mutation, abnormal cysts, and cancer.

Isn't she too young?

Teenagers or college-age girls often request the pill and are not always using it strictly for contraception. Sometimes, young women want the pill to help with their acne or cramps, while their parents feel that providing their daughters with oral contraceptives is like giving them a license to develop a wild sex life. Others worry about the long-term negative effects of the pill.

Relax. The pill doesn't make young women raging nymphomaniacs. In fact, behavior off and on the pill is very similar. So if you are having sex, you're better off on the pill, and if you're not having sex, you get some short-term help with your skin and cramps. Additionally, since you're bleeding less, you're less likely to be anemic or develop any kind of pelvic infection. Because your ovaries are less active,

vaginas

82

you're far less likely to develop ovarian disease, or endometriosis. And of course, for a young woman with a raging hormonal load and social calendar, one cannot underestimate the value of an even-keeled disposition and the ability to predict your period. And no, the birth control pill does not cause any long-term ill effects.

What if I get pregnant and continue taking the pill?
The pill is a sex hormone, so theoretically, all sorts of confusing gender things could happen with pregnancy. But over the course of the last fifty years, we've carefully observed women who didn't know they were pregnant and continued taking the pill. Not one birth defect has ever occurred that was attributable to the birth control pill. In retrospect, we suspect that the hormones in the pill are like a grain of sand on the beach of all the hormones a pregnant woman is making. Of course, if you are on the pill and learn that you are pregnant, discontinue taking it.

What's the difference between brands, and how do I know which is best for me?
With birth control pills and probably with almost everything, marketing is the big distinguishing factor between brands. This is not to say that there aren't minor differences between pills, but rather that no other person can know for you personally what the best choice is. If at first you don't succeed, try, try again.

One interesting new brand called Seasonal is the same birth control pill of old packaged differently. Instead of three weeks worth of active pills followed by one week of placebo, Seasonal has twelve weeks of active pills followed by one week of placebo. This presentation makes it easy to only have your period four times each year.

Why a twenty-eight day menstrual cycle? Do I have to have my period at all?
Recall that the menstrual cycle is defined as the period of time between the first day of your period to the first day of your next period. Twenty-

contraception

83

eight days is about average. However, there is no medical necessity to get your period when you're on the pill. Because you're taking both estrogen and progesterone every day, the lining of your uterus is never overstimulated (as it would be in a normal cycle or with estrogen alone) and it is not medically necessary to shed the endometrium. You can take these dual hormone active pills continuously and indefinitely and do no harm. Sooner or later, though, most women will break through and have a little vaginal bleeding. Stop taking the pill for no more than seven days (or you might ovulate) and then start over again.

Of course, missed periods in a woman who is not on the pill are concerning, and may signal hormonal disturbances, overexercising, undereating, stress, or a number of other ailments.

Which pill is good for my skin and why?
Most pills are good for your skin, but to be able to claim anything on the product label, the FDA requires that the manufacturer prove it. In other words, while almost all pills do help acne, the first company that actually went to the trouble of proving it was Ortho Tri-Cyclen.

Regardless, your first month on the pill your skin could be worse before it's better. All the pimples tend to come at the beginning of a hormone shift, so give it some time. It would be appropriate and fair to give a pill a three-month trial before you decide that it's not doing you or your skin any good.

BARRIER METHODS

Barrier contraceptive methods operate on a much more simple principal than the systemic hormonal treatments; they simply prevent the sperm from meeting the egg.

CONDOMS

The best overall contraceptive method is the condom, because although you pick up a slightly increased pregnancy rate, you earn a dramatically reduced infection rate. Not only do condoms prevent the sperm from meeting the egg, but they prevent the ejaculate from get-ting into your vagina and on your cervix. Most sexually transmitted diseases reside in semen, so it's best to avoid it. Condoms help to pre-vent transmission of the handful of STDs that can be transmitted through the skin (e.g. herpes and warts) because his genital skin never touches yours. That said, you should never, ever have sex under any conditions with someone who is having a herpes outbreak—condoms or not, herpes outbreaks are extremely contagious.

As great as they are, remember that condoms form a barrier against many but reduce your risk against all. In other words, condoms don't mean safe sex, but saf*er* sex. When a penis goes in a vagina, women catch things. Men too.

There are a lot of good things about a condom. It can be bought over the counter, so there's no excuse not to have one. If he's that hot to trot, he should be willing to go get a condom (or vice versa). It's dis-posable. One size fits many. It is technically easy to use. There are no side effects or risks of any kind.

There are many different kinds of condoms: latex, polyurethane, animal membrane, with the reservoir tip and without. Latex condoms with a reservoir tip are your best option. Polyurethane condoms are good for people with latex allergies. Animal membrane condoms are a nice, natural concept, but they do not protect against STDs—so this particular type is only recommended for people in a monogamous rela-tionship who are both disease free.

The condom was invented by the Marquis De Sade, who tied cheese-cloth at the base of his penis with a little bow. He didn't give a damn about getting a woman pregnant, but was very interested in protecting himself from infection. Rumor has it that he also invented the diaphragm, using half of a lemon (this is unverified). Perhaps this was an early attempt at combating an unpalatable smell.

Even latex condoms aren't perfect. In a recent study small holes were found in 10 percent of surgical gloves. Many surgeons now double-glove, which has significantly reduced infection rates. But if gloves used in an operating room have holes in them, it's logical to assume that condoms have plenty of holes as well. The concern here isn't pregnancy, which is reversible, as much as disease, which may not be.

We know that condoms have a somewhat unsexy reputation. Men have been heard to say, "It is like taking a shower with your raincoat on." Others say it's such a turn off that they can't maintain an erection over the course of putting a condom on (unimaginative whiners!). Meanwhile, some women feel that it looks premeditated and trampy for them to have condoms in their bedside table.

These are small issues in the face of what could be, quite frankly, a life or death situation. If you are having sex with someone outside of an ongoing monogamous relationship, if you're in a new relationship or if the two of you don't even have a relationship, you would have to be crazy not to use a condom.

Think of it as a new toy. Learn how to put them on with your mouth. There are all sorts of condoms—lubricated and unlubricated, ribbed, pink, flavored, etc. Get sexy with them. Challenge yourself to use them creatively and you just might have a good time.

The British have been known to call condoms, the *French letter*. Across the channel, they're called the *British hood*.

THE DIAPHRAGM

A much less effective form of barrier protection is the diaphragm. It looks like a rubber yarmulke, comes in different sizes, and is fitted in such a way as to wedge behind the pubic bone in your vagina and against the sacrum so that it snugly covers the cervix. As you might imagine, you need to have your diaphragm professionally fitted. The idea is to keep the sperm on the outside of the diaphragm, the egg on the other, and they can't meet.

You can insert your diaphragm with spermicide up to two hours before you have sex, but the closer you are to having sex, the more effective it will be because the spermicide does a good amount of the work. Less than two hours is an optimal amount of time. After sex, you have to leave it in for at least six hours, until all the little sperm lose their gusto.

Unfortunately, this is not a great way to avoid pregnancy. In perfect use situations, there is a 6 percent failure rate. In actual use, with spermicide applied before each encounter, the pregnancy rate is 20 percent. During sex, your vagina becomes swollen and dilated. In this changed environment, the diaphragm bobs all over the place. If you size it to fit as snugly as it would fit during sex, then it would be very painful for the six hours you have to wait before you remove it. Another unappealing feature is that diaphragm wearers have more frequent bladder infections.

contraception

87

...among many other contributions to women's reproductive advances, she brought the diaphragm to the United States from Europe in the early 1900s, risking her personal freedom. It was a crime to dispense any contraceptive device or advice, so she was arrested. Here was a woman who understood the significance of birth control.

SPERMICIDE

Spermicide is another form of nonhormonal, local contraception and is pretty self-explanatory. Nonoxynol 9 (the major ingredient in spermicide) kills the little sperm before they can implant in the egg. There are over-the-counter foams, creams, suppositories, and dozens of spermicidal preparations that a woman can buy without a doctor's prescription. The idea is to get the spermicide as close to the cervix as possible, where it is only effective for a limited amount of time (usually six hours). So with the sponge, for example, it's good for six hours, then you have to wait six hours, so that's six hours you're definitely not having sex.

You can find spermicide in your local drug store, right next to all the waxing stuff, tampons, etc. usually secreted away in the "woman's corner." If you are an over-the-counter kind of person who is monogamous and therefore don't have to worry as much about STDs, then using spermicide once per day is probably okay.

WARNING

As stated in the Condom section, a recent study suggests that spermicide increases your risk of infection by compromising your epithelium (i.e. it irritates your skin, which makes it easier for infections to enter your bloodstream). Current guidelines suggest limiting your use of spermicide to once per day. More than that may increase your risk of contracting HIV.

CERVICAL CAP

You've probably never heard of the cervical cap—a small, rigid, rubber device much like the diaphragm—held on the cervix by suction. The truth is that if Margaret Sanger had met the cervical cap distributor before she met the diaphragm representative in Europe, then women in America would probably have cervical caps and the diaphragm would be a fringe option.

Or maybe not. The cervical cap is rather difficult to use. Back in the 1930s, women would go to the doctor right after their periods to get the cap put on and come back right before their periods to get it taken off. Not only was this inconvenient, but as Pap smears became more and more accurate, we noticed a significant increase in abnormal Pap smears for cervical cap wearers. This is not to say that the cap increased incidence of disease, but led to more atypical cells and inflammation.

As women seized the reins of their reproductive health, they clamored for more contraceptive options, and the cervical cap was among the temporary darlings of the women's movement. But without the aid of a doctor, the cervical cap can be a bitch to use, and 20 percent of women cannot use them at all—they just won't fit.

Despite the fact that cervical caps were never widely used, there are a few current options if the description above sounds good to you. The only cap presently available in the United States is called FemCap. Rather than suck onto your cervix, it stabilizes itself on the walls of the

Cervical Caps Meet Pristine Cervixes

One of the largest hurdles for the cervical cap aficionados is finding the right size. Up until the sexual revolution, contraception was geared towards married women who had already finished with reproduction, not single women. With each baby that you deliver vaginally, your cervix permanently swells (like most women's waistlines). Caps were targeted at these women, so they are often too big for women who never had children.

vagina. Lea's Shield is the brand name of another new cap that may soon become available in the States. There could be a few women out there who love their little rubber caps, but there are so many more effective, easier options, I find it hard to suggest the cap to anyone seeking contraception.

THE IUD

The Intrauterine Device (or IUD) is the most effective, inexpensive form of reversible contraception. IUDs are small, usually T-shaped devices that accommodate the shape of the uterus, where they are placed by a physician. Usually IUD insertion happens around the time of your period, when menstruation has caused the cervix to dilate slightly. This makes it easier for a gynecologist to insert a foreign body into your uterus. By significantly disrupting the environment of the uterus (and blocking the path of those eager sperm), the IUD prevents the fertilized egg from implanting. The part of the uterus that the IUD irritates gets shed every month, without affecting or irritating the uterus itself.

The IUD as contraceptive device has been through many stages on its way to being the safe, effective option it is today. At the turn of the last century, inserting an IUD was irreversible, rendering women (generally who had finished building their families) permanently sterile. These devices were occasionally made of jewel-encrusted gold and went to the grave with their owners. Today, the FDA and the medical establishment require that the instrument be removable.

Also, the device has to be easy to insert and have a documented effectiveness rate. IUDs are statistically as effective as surgical sterilization, at a 0.6 percent pregnancy rate. We've also addressed many of the early problems with IUDs, and only recommend them to women who are mutually monogamous and want long-term contraception. One of the things to bear in mind with IUDs is that they do not prevent ectopic pregnancies, so if you are an IUD wearer and experience extreme pelvic pain, that might be the first thing an emergency room doctor should look for.

∙∙∙

The story goes that camel drivers in the Middle East would put rocks inside female camel uteri so that they wouldn't get pregnant on long caravans, and therefore require more water. This was reputed to be the origin of the IUD. While it is a cool story, it has never been verified, and at last check, no actual camel driver had ever heard of this technique.

∙∙∙

While the fear with IUDs used to be Pelvic Inflammatory Disease (PID), current information suggests that IUDs do not increase the rate of PID. Monogamous IUD wearers have less than a 1 percent risk of infection because they and their partner's flora grow to be very much the same. It's kind of romantic, actually, as you share a bed you become one ecosystem. His penis is full of nice, familiar bacteria.

There are two IUDs available today—the copper T or Paragard T and a progesterone-releasing IUD called the Levonorgesterel-releasing intrauterine system or, for short, Mirena. The progesterone IUD is not marketed as an IUD, but as a delivery system for the progesterone, which alters the mucus so the sperm can't swim effectively. Like all IUDs, Mirena also alters the lining of the uterus so that the endometrium is hostile to a possible embryo. Progesterone is a relaxant, so it diminishes the traditional problems of cramps and bleeding during the period. Twenty percent of women using Mirena stop menstruating after one year. The progesterone IUD lasts five years. The advantage of the copper "T" is that it lasts ten years, but it can cause increased cramps and bleeding. Should you go past the approved time limit for either, you have a slightly increased risk of pregnancy.

The IUD just might be making a comeback, because it is as effective as anything and it doesn't require remembering to take a pill or insert a ring. While there is the small possibility that you'll react badly to an IUD—experience discomfort, cramping, spotting—with the progesterone IUD there's also a 20 percent chance you will cease menstruating after one year until you remove the device.

The Dalkon Shield was probably the saddest singular casualty on our march towards reproductive freedom. The Dalkon Shield was an IUD that looked a little bit like a turtle; it was a triangular shaped plastic device with little spigots sticking out all around it. The string that extended into the vagina for easy extraction was a polyfilmant (it was braided). This device was distributed to the public after an extremely brief and probably inadequate trial.

It turned out that the strings they chose to use, for most IUDs but the Dalkon Shield in particular, served as a transport medium between the outside world of the vagina and the inside of these poor women's uteri. Many young women with IUDs got high temperatures, pelvic infections, and abscesses. The problem with the Dalkon Shield, which had the highest rate of infection, was the braided string, which rapidly wicked the bacteria in the vagina up into the uterus.

This led to a significant increase in pelvic infections, as many unmonogamous young women were getting Dalkon Shields and other IUDs. Within a year of the Shield's introduction, there were women who had become pregnant despite their IUDs and died. As their pregnancies progressed, the device would be drawn up into the uterus, causing fatal infections.

It may be hard to understand how such oversights could have happened, but in the sixties, a lot of energy was focused on family planning and contraception. Women were rightfully becoming more politically active, so the FDA was under pressure to provide as many options as possible. Many women were given IUDs without any consideration of their lifestyle, age, or reproductive desires. And we quickly learned that a woman with multiple sexual partners was at great risk for a severe pelvic infection if she used an IUD, because she was exposing herself to lots of different bacteria that would be carried up via the IUD into her uterus.

NATURAL FAMILY PLANNING
(FORMERLY KNOWN AS THE "RHYTHM" METHOD)

The idea with natural family planning is to figure out when you ovulate each month and avoid having sex around those times. As there are plenty of theoretical and actual signs for ovulation, it's easy to figure out when ovulation happened and have sex afterward and through the next period. It is much more difficult to gauge the safe interval between the period and a projected ovulation date.

There are plenty of ovulation flags. If you're willing to examine your cervix every day by inserting a finger and touching it, you'll notice that it gets softer after you ovulate. You can also examine your cervical mucus every day. When it turns creamy, you've ovulated. In addition, your temperature goes up after you've ovulated because progesterone is hyperthermic (it raises your body temperature). You can use an ovulation predictor kit, which at twenty dollars a pop can get costly after your third test each month. These kits can target between twelve and thirty-six hours before ovulation. If you're trying to get pregnant, this would be a good time to go for it. If you're trying to avoid pregnancy, you have seventy-two hours to wait before the egg perishes and you can resume sexual activity. There are also pocket computers that can help to predict your fertile and infertile times if you can't be bothered to keep a close eye on the calendar or your cervix.

Menstrual cycles vary. If you have really regular periods (and predicting your period should never be something you bet a whole lot

contraception

93

I remember this couple in college who were very in love but very religious. She told me that they took turns policing their sexual activity. One focused on stopping and the other relaxed and enjoyed whatever they were doing. The minute it looked like his penis was getting too close to her vagina, whosever turn it was would say, "Okay, stop!" She wanted to be a virgin on her wedding night.

of money on), you ovulate around day fourteen of a twenty-eight day cycle. Therefore, you should probably stop at least one week prior to ovulation. So you can have unprotected regular intercourse during your period and up to seven days afterwards. Then you can have unprotected intercourse three days after ovulation through your period and to day seven again. That's eighteen out of twenty-eight days to play with.

The more days you abstain around ovulation, the more effective this method is. There are very disciplined people who have intercourse two or three days a month and guess what? No pregnancy. But the human mind is a funny thing—you keep cutting down on your abstinent days and eventually you get pregnant. You either need to be very disciplined or, on the days that you say, "Aw, screw it," use a condom. I know many a woman who's had an unexpected baby using natural family planning, and many others who have never had any surprises.

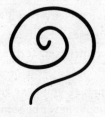

COITUS INTERRUPTUS

The most shaky of all contraception is coitus interruptus with an estimated 20 percent pregnancy rate. Here the man "pulls out" just before he ejaculates, preventing most of the semen from entering the vagina. This is not a great option for those of you who really do not want to get pregnant. It's not something that I would count on, but if you're reading this book and have been practicing coitus interruptus without any slipups for ten years, then keep on keeping on.

TUBAL LIGATION

Also known as "having your tubes tied," tubal ligation is the most widely used contraceptive method in the United States. At a pregnancy rate of 0.5 to 3.5 percent, it's extremely effective, and can be very cost effective if done at a point when the patient has a sizeable number of fertile years left. The procedure takes about thirty minutes, and you can leave the hospital the same day. Some women are back to work after two days, while others take two weeks to recover—this is entirely dependent on the patient's comfort level. The two significant negatives of this procedure are that it's surgery and carries the risk of general anesthesia (one in ten thousand people die) and that it is considered permanent.

Advances in reproductive technology have made it possible for women who have had a tubal ligation to still become biological mothers. A fertility specialist can harvest your eggs, bypassing the tube, and

Contraception in Italy

Some say the number one form of contraception in Italy is anal intercourse. I don't want to get sued by the country that I love more than anyplace, but this has some logic to it. You're still a virgin, you're definitely not going to get pregnant, and you might be having fun.

implant a fertilized egg in your uterus. This comes at considerable expense of time, money, and energy. So it's a good idea to be absolutely certain that your childbearing is behind you before you have this operation.

There are a number of ways to tie your tubes, and your doctor probably has her favorite. The Pommeroy procedure is most often used in addition to an abdominal surgery, like at the time of a caesarian section. Here, the surgeon clamps both tubes (they're like giant, hollow, cooked spaghetti), folds them in half, ties them with a suture, and cuts the loops off. The sutures are biodegradable, and once dissolved, the patient is left with two big gaps in the middle of the fallopian tubes. The sperm stops at one scarred patch, and across a vast chasm, the egg is stuck on the other side.

It is also possible to do tubal ligations laproscopically (a tiny medical device involving cameras and lasers), which involves a much smaller incision through the belly button. In this procedure, the surgeon burns the middle part of the tube to achieve the same result. The advantages to this procedure are that it is usually better tolerated by the patient, allowing her to return more quickly to full activity, and it produces a nearly invisible scar. This is becoming the number one method of tubal ligation, especially for women who have no need for another abdominal operation.

God bless you if you can and if you want to.

A BRIEF AND SUBJECTIVE RETROSPECTIVE
ON TUBAL LIGATION

Tubal ligation was developed as a quick way to permanently sterilize a woman while allowing her to get back to work almost immediately. It does not require a lot of time or a great amount of medical expertise. No surprise then that tubal ligation was developed in the concentration camps of Nazi Germany.

There was a lot of mythology around tubal ligation when I was in medical school. In Puerto Rico, there was the misconception that if you got your tubes tied, you'd be fertile again after five years. Many mothers brought their wayward daughters in for this procedure, and then thought I was trying to withhold this five-year magic contraceptive from them. I also saw many women who had had their tubes tied six years prior and wondered why they couldn't get pregnant.

When I was in Jamaica in the 1970s, women were very reluctant to have their tubes tied, because there was the theory of "allotment." This superstition dictates that women are fated to have a certain number of children, and to tamper with fate is to invite a curse on yourself. The professionals I spoke to felt this was a throwback to the days of slavery, when the healthcare providers to the slave community were in the pay of slave owners, and therefore likely to encourage as many children as possible. So Jamaican women felt very negative about any limitation whatsoever on their reproductive function, permanent ones most especially.

Like hysterectomies (see page 216), attitudes and methods of tubal ligation vary from country to country, and within the United States, from region to region. This has a lot to do with when women begin and end their childbearing, as well as the relative ease of the pro-

contraception

97

We believe we've covered all the legitimate contraceptive measures. Forget practices like douching right after intercourse, jumping up and down after sex, the last minute condom, or the idea that if you didn't have an orgasm you can't get pregnant. If that last one were true, the Baby Boom would have been more like a baby blip.

cedure. I had a patient who was visiting her dying father in the Minnesota, and wound up in the emergency room with an ectopic pregnancy. She was scared, upset, and sleep deprived. The hospital doctor said, "We think we have to operate—we think it's an ectopic. But, as long as we're in there, would you like us to tie the other tube?" She was about thirty-five. While most women still start their families in their twenties, thirty-five (which is far older than the national average) is when many of my patients commence childbearing. She told the doctor, "Do what you have to do." He took that as consent and tied her other tube.

The sad irony was that she came to me several years later because she was having trouble getting pregnant. This doctor thought he was doing her a great favor. Needless to say, when she found out he had tied her other tube, she was shocked.

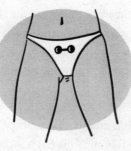

		PREGNANCY RATES	STD PROTECTION	COST	RX	ITEMS OF NOTE
"Oral" contraceptives i.e. estrogen & progesterone combined	Pill	0.5 % Perfect Use* 3% Typical Use	NONE	Variable; approximately $30/month	Y	You have to remember to take a pill every day. The newest wrinkles: Ortho Tri-Cyclen— Good for Acne Yasmin — Good for Bloating Seasonal — Four periods per year
	Ortho Evra (Skin Patch)	0.5% Perfect Use 3% Typical Use	NONE	More than the Pill	Y	Less effective if you're over 200 lbs. Change the patch weekly. Some women report skin irritation.
	Nuva (Vaginal Ring)	0.5% Perfect Use 3% Typical Use	NONE	Aproximately $50/month	Y	You only have to remember once a month to take it out, wait a week and put a new one in. One size fits all.

*Perfect use is the theoretical maximum efficacy. However, in our day-to-day lives, we forget, in our day-to-day lives, we forget, we drift within four hours of our usual time, etc. Hence the higher pregnancy rate. The World Health Organization (WHO) calculates pregnancy rates in women/years. Which means that out of a hundred women in a year using a particular method of contraception, how many get pregnant.

		PREGNANCY RATES	STD PROTECTION	COST	RX	ITEMS OF NOTE
	Lunelle (Monthly injection)	0.5% Perfect Use 3% Typical Use	NONE	Not out yet	Y	You have to go to the doctor's office once each month for your shot. Currently being reformatted.
Progesterone only	Pill	0.3% Perfect Use 8% Typical Use	NONE	Variable; approximately $30/month	Y	Will not suppress lactation.
	Depo Provera	0.3% Perfect Use 3% Typical Use	NONE	$100 every three months	Y	Will not suppress lactation. Injection every three months. Popular with teenagers. 9,000,000 women worldwide. Often suppresses menstruation.

		PREGNANCY RATES	STD PROTECTION	COST	RX	ITEMS OF NOTE
	Levonorgestrel-releasing intrauterine system (IUD)	0.1 – 0.2%	NONE	Approximately $1000	Y	Will not suppress lactation. Nothing to think about. Good for five years. 20% of women don't get their period at all. Good for assorted gynecological menstrual problems. Same pregnancy rate as tubal ligation but reversible. MUST be monogamous.
Subdermal Implanet	Implanon, Norplant, Norplant-2	0.05%	NONE	N/A	Y	Not available in the United States.
IUD	Paragard T	0.6%	NONE	$800	Y	Good for ten years. May increase cramps and bleeding.
	Levonorgestrel-releasing intrauterine system (IUD)	See Above	See Above	See Above		See Above.

		PREGNANCY RATES	STD PROTECTION	COST	RX	ITEMS OF NOTE
Barriers	**Condom (male)**	3% Perfect Use 14% Typical Use	Very Good	+-1$ EACH	N	This is the method of choice for non-monogamous people. Avoid natural condoms—use latex only, unless monogamous.
	Condom (female)	5% Perfect Use 21% Typical Use	Excellent	+-$3 EACH	N	Probably the best way to protect yourself from STDs. I've never seen one and don't know anyone who's ever used one.
	Diaphragm	6% Perfect Use 20% Typical Use	NONE	$20 Plus Doctor's fee	Y	Increased risk of bladder and vaginal infections. Inconvenient. God bless you, Margaret Sanger, but she'd be the first to move on.
	Cervical Cap	9% Perfect Use 40% Typical Use	NONE	$20	Y	Difficult to use. Seems to cause abnormal Pap smears.

	PREGNANCY RATES	STD PROTECTION	COST	RX	ITEMS OF NOTE
Spermicide	6% Perfect Use 26% Typical Use	NONE	VARIES	N	Nonoxynol-9 has recently been linked to increased infection rates, especially HIV and with frequent use. Nonoxynol-9 coated condoms are no longer recommended.
The Sponge	9% to 40%	NONE	VARIES	N	Pregnancy rates for The Sponge increase dramatically after a vaginal delivery.
Natural Family Planning **Rhythm**	19% to 25%	NONE	FREE	N	The more days you abstain, the higher your contraceptive efficacy. Good Luck!
Coitus Interruptus	?	NONE	FREE	N	I have plenty of patients who use this method and have never gotten pregnant, but I wouldn't count on it.
Surgery **Tubal Ligation**	0.5 – 3.5%	NONE	VARIES but up to several thousand dollars	Y	#1 contraceptive method in the U.S.A. This method carries a mortality rate because it is surgery—1 in 10,000 women die. #1 complication is regret.

MOTHER: "When I was in college, all the liberated girls went right to the health service and got a diaphragm."

DAUGHTER: "So you had a diaphragm in college?"

MOTHER: "I was a late bloomer."

DAUGHTER: "Did you ever have a diaphragm?"

MOTHER: "For about three days."

DAUGHTER: "Why was that?"

MOTHER: "Well, you know your father. Leave him alone for five minutes and he falls asleep. So I'd excuse myself and by the time I got back he'd be snoring."

DAUGHTER: "Talk about something I didn't want to know...."

chapter seven

SEXUALLY TRANSMITTED DISEASES

These days, we hear "AIDS epidemic" and think, Africa. During my time in southern and eastern Africa, the disease was both omnipresent and eerily absent. There are scattered visible efforts at public health awareness, and in some places, you can forget about the problem entirely; until someone lightly remarks on their own positive HIV status. Funeral homes dot the townships outside of Johannesburg like the Gap on New York City streets. Pictures of young people stack the obituaries, the listings discreetly citing "long illness" as the cause of their deaths. Street children—most of them AIDS orphans—in small gangs follow tourists begging. In the bazaars, stalls display fake funeral flower arrangements made out of colorful, discarded plastic bags. The worst may be over in the Western world, but in Africa it is still to come.

Before we get into the specifics of sexually transmitted infections, let's try to discard the cultural and social stigmas attached to this subset of illness. These are diseases like any other, and you should not feel your dignity is compromised because you are sick.

Any disease usually transmitted through sex is a sexually transmitted disease, though almost any infectious illness can be caught through sexual contact and almost any STD can be caught from nonsexual behavior. Think of a common cold, for example. If you have sex with someone who has a bad cold, you're probably going to catch it, but we don't think of colds as STDs because you could catch them through much more casual contact. On the other hand, if you have a cold sore on your lip, you touch it, and then scratch your genitals, you may have just given yourself genital herpes.

There are around twenty-five known STDs. Luckily for us North Americans, the majority of STDs are tropical, meaning those particular bacteria are so fastidious, they can't survive in colder climates. There are also some diseases that haven't hit us as hard in the north, due to a prevalence of monogamy and safe sex practices. All STDs fall into three groups: bacterial, viral, and parasitic.

BACTERIAL STDS

GONORRHEA AND CHLAMYDIA

The good news about bacteria is that we can treat them very effectively. The bad news is that 75 to 80 percent of women with gonorrhea or chlamydia are asymptomatic. Things to be on the lookout for are burning when urinating or a pussy penile/vaginal discharge. In women, these symptoms suggest a strong possibility of bacterial infection. In men, these symptoms specifically signify gonorrhea or chlamydia until proven otherwise.

Gonorrhea and chlamydia are detectable within three to six days of exposure. Usually a cervical culture will pick it up. Once diagnosed, we prescribe antibiotics. However, since these infections can keep a low profile, diagnosis can be tricky and if unchecked, they can develop into a painful and fertility-threatening problem.

If you have unprotected sex with a man who has gonorrhea or chlamydia, the bacteria piggybacks on the semen and gets deposited right onto the cervix, which is a very friendly environment to them. Sooner or later, you get your period, and the bacteria thrive on the blood, feasting and reproducing. When your period ceases, the little bugs head up to the uterus and out into the tubes searching for more food. The hungry bacteria damage the fallopian tubes as they travel upward, causing scarring and sometimes closing the end of the tubes nearest the ovaries.

The condition that eventually develops is called Pelvic Inflammatory Disease (PID), which the residents at my hospital cutely call "pusindere" (pus in there). This is the name we use for any infection that affects the ovary and fallopian tubes. It can be excruciatingly painful and unnecessarily tragic. If the bacteria are not immediately treated, or are treated incompletely, the damage to the tubes can lead to scarring and infertility (see page 206).

Go to your doctor and get a vaginal culture if you have a new partner and practice unsafe sex. If you get a call from a sexual partner who says, "I think I have an infection. It burns when I urinate," take the call seriously (thank him!) and act quickly. You can't wait a week or two until you have time, because in the interim, bacteria could be doing significant harm to your reproductive organs. At the very least, call your doctor immediately. For a woman who wants to have babies, this is as important as any doctor's appointment you'll ever make.

SYPHILIS

Syphilis starts as a sore about two weeks after contact. This is sometimes overlooked because it can come and go very quickly. Then, several weeks later, secondary syphilis causes a blotchy, flat, red rash. The characteristic uniqueness with this stage is that it affects the palms of your hands and the soles of your feet (where most rashes do not grow). For this reason, up until the 1980s, syphilis was diagnosed and treated by dermatologists.

Spirochetes

Lyme disease and syphilis are both caused by odd, spiral-shaped bacteria. They're both great imitators of other diseases, and have the ability to lodge in a wide variety of places. Depending on where they choose to stick, they can give you a spectrum of vague symptoms, such as swollen glands, anemia, and a flulike syndrome in the early stages, to intellectual deterioration and necrotic ulcers if the disease continues unchecked.

After the rash stage, the spirochetes find a place to live—in muscle, in the brain, or in the nerves. No one knows how long it can remain dormant, because at this point, the disease has either been diagnosed and cured, or it eventually progresses onto the final stage, so no one was tracking it from the beginning. Once the bacteria has moved in, the patient can appear to be in perfectly fine health for up to twenty years before she comes down with tertiary syphilis. This is a very nasty, irreversible development. Tertiary syphilis can damage your organs, including the nervous system, heart, or brain to the point of institutionalization. But you have plenty of time to treat this problem before it becomes life threatening.

Sometimes a syphilis-related aneurysm can compress one of the nerves next to the vocal chords, forcing the sufferer to speak in a husky whisper. This condition was called "prostitutes' whisper" in the fourteenth century. Suffice it to say, if you frequent ladies of the night, try to avoid the ones with hoarse voices.

Syphilis is commonly tested for and easy to treat. Every time you have surgery, and up to twice when you are pregnant, you will be given a blood test for syphilis. Syphilis can be cured with penicillin, so if you contract and identify it within a reasonable amount of time, it's not something to worry about. It is, however, dangerous for pregnant women because the disease can spread to the child, causing birth defects and an increased risk of stillbirth.

VIRUSES

Viruses can be treated but not medically cured. In other words, we can't prescribe something to kill the virus the way we can kill bacteria, but your body has its own defense in antibodies. With some viruses, like measles, you completely recover and become immune for the rest of your life. With others, the virus remains in your body forever.

HERPES

Herpes is one of the most infamous of all viruses, and it's unfortunately very, very contagious. Herpes is one of the relatively few STDs that can be transmitted from skin to skin contact.

After you've been exposed, the incubation period is two to twenty-one days, meaning you will develop a lesion within that period if you've caught the virus. The virus family of which herpes is a member likes to live on and affect nerve roots, which means within the incu-

sexually transmitted diseases

109

In the 1930s, a group of scientists set out to determine whether syphilis behaves the same in Caucasian and African American patients. They observed a group of black men with syphilis for decades, long after penicillin came out. The unfortunate subjects of the experiment were allowed to progress to tertiary symptoms, including death and brain damage. This is one of the great blights on our medical history. Today, we don't continue clinical studies after we've discovered a cure or realize that we are doing harm.

bation period, you will frequently have neurological symptoms—e.g. pain down the leg, pain in the pelvis, or even general aches and pains. The nerves to the bladder can be affected and make it hard to pee. The virus circulates through your bloodstream, which leads to flulike symptoms or a sense of malaise—patients typically say they feel like they're "coming down with something." This is your first or primary outbreak and is usually the worst one you'll experience.

There are exceptions to this rule, however. If you are particularly healthy, you may not have symptoms when you have caught the herpes virus. Then a year or two later, you get run down or stressed out, and you have what appears to be your primary outbreak.

The worst part of the virus for most people are the lesions. They start off looking like a blister, then the bubble bursts, and they become an open sore. Usually, these last seven to ten days and fade away. To repeat, the first outbreak is generally the worst, potentially producing multiple sores all over the vagina, labia, cervix, and rectum, and painful swollen glands in the groin.

A major symptom of viruses or any infection in your genitalia is swollen glands in your groin. Glands filter out any foreign bodies from your blood stream. For example, whenever there's a break in the skin and bacteria gets in, the lymph nodes drain dangerous germs before

Return to Bio 101— A Technical Introduction to Viruses

Viruses are intracellular organisms, meaning they live within healthy cells and co-opt parts of their host's DNA to perform vital metabolic functions, such as reproduction. This means that viral cells cannot live for very long without a healthy host cell. Testing for viruses is tricky, because they're quite happy to live inside your cells, which camouflage them. The most common way to test for viruses is to test for antibodies—your body's natural defense against a viral assault. After thriving inside a host, the viral cells increase in quantity, and the host cell explodes. The freed viral cells search for new hosts, and the process begins all over again on a larger scale.

they get to the heart. The glands in the groin are responsible for removing all unwanted and dangerous material from the external genitalia and the legs. If you feel lumps in your groin, like swollen olive pits, this could be a sign of a virus, like herpes (or that you got your legs waxed).

Once you've been diagnosed, an immediate blood test can distinguish between a primary and recurrent outbreak; the patient will either have antibodies to herpes, or there will be a rise in antibodies two weeks later. If she already has the antibodies at the time of what she thinks is her first outbreak, it is definitely a recurrent infection. And if

Herpes I, Herpes II

When the herpes virus was first identified, they distinguished between herpes I (oral) and herpes II (genital). You may not realize that cold sores, canker sores, or any really nasty, painful lesion in your mouth is probably herpes. Thanks to oral sex, these days plenty of herpes I reside in the genitals, and herpes II is found in many a mouth. This difference is mostly academic, and generally diagnosed by location as opposed to a specific type.

sexually transmitted diseases

I once had a particularly young, independent ballerina as a patient. She was about sixteen. She came in with her first herpes outbreak, and I prescribed a medicine to help keep her very significant symptoms in check. The next day, her boyfriend called me to ask why I had prescribed that particular medication, as the last two women he had slept with had been given something different. I asked him what the Hell he thought he was doing, and he said, "Well, doc, a guy's gotta live."

there's any doubt that the genital lesions are herpes, a swab of the sore will almost definitely determine whether it's the big H or not.

It's only important to distinguish between primary and secondary outbreaks for two reasons. First, a primary outbreak during pregnancy can be very serious, as the virus can cross the placenta and cause complications. A recurrent outbreak does not endanger the baby. Second, most people want to know, if possible, where they picked up the virus. Married people are usually particularly "curious."

Once you have herpes, recurrences can be anywhere from extraordinarily infrequent (never) to very frequent (twice a month). This is directly related to your emotional and physical well-being. Stress of all kinds can be an invitation for an outbreak, as it weakens your immune system. If your immune system is already not so hot, you're at greater risk for outbreaks. However, as long as your immunity is not clinically compromised (as it is for newborn babies, people on chemotherapy and with AIDS), your life is not endangered.

REMEMBER

Never never never have sex with someone who has a herpes outbreak — condom or not, this is an incredibly contagious virus when you're dealing with open sores.

Treatment

We've come a long way in controlling herpes, although there is no cure. There are antiviral medications in various strengths (e.g. Zovarax, Valtrex, and Famvir), which come in high and low dose pills or intravenously for immune-compromised people. High dosage pills are for acute intervention, generally for those terrible first outbreaks. Sometimes doctors will also prescribe topical Zovarax, which is less effective than systemic treatments, but it helps. For severe recurrent outbreaks, especially if they are infrequent, a short course of a high dosage pill will help. For very frequent outbreaks, usually more than six a year, patients can take a low dose pill every day to prevent outbreaks from happening. After a year of constant medication, patients frequently reduce the dose to the bare minimum that is still effective.

Pregnancy is Not the Time for Secrets

I've had a few pregnant patients with herpes. One came in with her husband when she was eight months pregnant. She had a funny lesion. I said, "This looks like herpes," and the husband turned green. He'd known all along and never told her. She found out about two weeks before she was delivering their first baby. I had another married, pregnant woman who had herpes, and under no circumstances was I allowed to tell her husband. I said, "What if you have an outbreak?" She told me I would just have to make up something. I said, "But he'll be there. He'll see that the baby is okay." Ultimately, I think we made up some reason for a section. But it was very difficult for all of us, and I don't think that maintaining this secret was very healthy for their relationship. It's scary and awkward to tell a partner about your STD, but no matter how terrible the reaction is, it's never as bad as you've imagined it. Tell the guy for God's sake! Think of it as test of his character. If he walks, he's not worth it.

Herpes and Pregnancy

The big concern with herpes is pregnancy. If there is an active lesion when the patient is in labor, the baby cannot be exposed to it on the way through the vagina. Among a host of physical ailments, herpes can damage the brain of a newborn. Should a pregnant patient have an outbreak at the time of delivery, there is no choice but to perform a Caesarian section. However, herpes is something your doctor should be well aware of before delivery. She would then be able to prescribe antivirals for about three weeks prior to the due date, preventing an outbreak and allowing for a vaginal delivery. This seems to be successful and therefore has solved what was a considerable issue in obstetrics.

HUMAN PAPILLOMA VIRUS (HPV)

Human Papilloma Virus is the most common of all sexually transmitted diseases and usually the most innocuous. Any wart on your body is caused by some strain of HPV and is contagious from skin to skin contact. Virtually all sexually active young adults have HPV at some point. As of 2004, HPV is considered to be a transient, relatively harmless virus for over 95 percent of young women. This means that your body will rid your system of the virus within three to five years, with no symptoms or ill affects.

There are almost a hundred identified strains of the virus, two small groups of which are cause for concern. The first group, called "low risk" strains, causes genital warts, which are unsightly but ultimately not dangerous. The second group, called "high risk" strains, causes cervical cancer, which is almost never fatal if detected and treated early enough, especially *before* it becomes cancer.

A few strains of low-risk HPV cause warts. Anyone who has had to sit through a high school sex education class knows that genital warts are among the most unsightly things that can happen to the human body. They grow indefinitely at unpredictable rates, and they're very contagious. We generally laser, freeze, or cut them off. If these options make your skin crawl, there are a few topical treatments that stimulate your natural defenses to fight the warts. After three to five years, the warts are

@vaginas

If you're an oncologist, HPV is a fascinating infection. HPV is the only virus we know of that causes tumors and cancer, and theoretically, we have a lot to learn from it. So far, the breakthroughs have been limited to effectively preventing cervical cancer. Currently, they're working on an HPV vaccine for the highest risk strains. Vaccines don't work if you've already been exposed, so this is something we might give to pre-adolescents in the future.

gone, your Pap should return to normal, and you're as healthy as anyone. There is often no HPV virus present in your system.

HPV is a necessary precursor to cervical cancer, and therefore, we can say that HPV causes cervical cancer. Approximately one-tenth of HPV strains are considered high-risk carcinogens.

Before Pap smears, cervical cancer was the number one genital cancer in this country, and it's still a serious problem in the developing world. Since most women in this country have access to at least occasional Pap smears, cervical cancer has fallen behind uterine and ovarian cancer as the most common gynecological cancers. See the chapter on Significant Problems of the Cervix (page 234) for more information on this disease and your treatment options.

HEPATITIS B

Hepatitis B is unique among STDs in that it is the only one that you can be vaccinated against. The vaccine consists of a series of shots, given some months apart.

Hepatitis B feels like a very bad flu. Early symptoms include extreme fatigue, fever, vomiting, a yellowing of the skin, dark urine, and light stool. For reasons unknown, smokers typically lose their taste for cigarettes when they have Hepatitis. Usually, this is as far as the disease progresses, and it lasts up to a few months. However, the illness attacks

sexually transmitted diseases

115

the liver, and in particularly bad cases, can lead to liver cancer and death. Approximately 10 percent of adults who contract Hepatitis B die.

There is no real treatment for Hepatitis B. Generally, we recommend bed rest, eating right, and patience for the duration of the illness. Once your body has beaten back the virus, you are no longer contagious. For a rare few, it becomes chronic. The virus lives in the victim's liver forever, causing symptoms that can be mild to severe, and eventually kills them. There are currently efforts to prevent liver damage for people with chronic Hepatitis B through medication.

Almost all babies in this country are now vaccinated within a few weeks of life against Hepatitis B. Hopefully, within our lifetimes, Hepatitis B will be like polio or bubonic plague—an extraordinarily, rare disease.

HUMAN IMMUNODEFICIENCY VIRUS (HIV) AND AUTOIMMUNE DEFICIENCY SYNDROME (AIDS)

While HIV and the illness that it leads to, AIDS have received more press than any STD since herpes, there are only a handful of people who can accurately explain how the virus works and the myriad treatment strategies.

A Personal Story

In my medical career I've only had one HIV test come back positive. Sadly, it was for David, my best friend since he took me to my junior prom. He had shared a beach house with about ten other homosexual men who had all passed away due to HIV-related complications. He was feeling rundown and losing weight. When he told me years before that he had broken up with a guy because he wanted to use a condom, I yelled and screamed at him but . . . it was the early nineties when he came to my office. I drew the blood, and a week later I went to his apartment to deliver the tragic news in person. Several years later, he passed away.

@vaginas

It's very difficult to tell what kind of sexual behavior carries the highest risk of transmission—i.e. very few people have sex without kissing. Physicians assume that the riskiest behavior involves the fluid that has the highest viral load, blood, and that the lowest risk involves no bodily fluid, like mutual masturbation or, even better, phone sex. Any break in the skin of either person leads to a higher risk situation. If you have gum disease, you give someone oral sex and they ejaculate into your mouth, the virus can get right into your bloodstream through the gums. If you have anal intercourse, and there is an abrasion or a laceration, then you are also at high risk. Play gently.

Recall from above that viral cells move into healthy cells, where they happily live and reproduce, until the cells get too crowded. The HIV virus lives in and ultimately attacks T-cells, which draw their name from the thymus gland where they mature. T-cells are one of many soldiers in the ranks of our complex immune system, primarily responsible for our resistance to a handful of diseases that were previously very rare or only found in the elderly. These are ailments that a healthy body (with healthy T-cells) can readily defeat.

With HIV and AIDS, therefore, the basic metric physicians use to determine your relative health is your T-cell count. Over three hundred is an adequate T-cell count, while people with full-blown AIDS can have a T-cell count as low as zero. Another test that is used in the management of HIV is a measure of how much virus there is in your system, called a viral load test. The higher the viral load, and the lower the T-cell count, the sicker you are.

The HIV virus is present in blood, semen, vaginal fluids, tears, saliva, and breast milk in relative amounts. Of all of these, blood has the highest viral concentration, while tears have the lowest. While we know it as an STD, HIV can also be transmitted from one IV drug user to

sexually transmitted diseases

I have several patients who have HIV, and several other patients whose husbands are HIV positive while they have remained negative. I have two patients who had healthy babies and remained healthy themselves with HIV-positive husbands. This is an expensive proposition, involving in vitro fertilization (in the United States) and/or specialized sperm-washing techniques and insemination (only done in Europe). These men have had the virus for twelve and eighteen years respectively, and they are both healthy.

another when they share a needle, or from an HIV-positive mother to her unborn or breast-feeding child. Approximately 30 percent of pregnant, HIV-positive women have HIV-positive babies. That risk is reduced to 7 percent if you receive treatment while pregnant. Therefore, New York State law mandates HIV testing for pregnant women, and if the mother has not been tested, the child will be upon delivery.

Transient flulike symptoms usually develop within several days of contracting HIV. This is often overlooked, as it comes and goes, and is usually only noticed retrospectively. Later symptoms include any seemingly unthreatening problem that just won't go away—like a persistent yeast infection that defies all treatments and lasts months and months.

To test for HIV, we look for antibodies that your body has naturally produced in response to the virus. These don't happen overnight, and it can take up to six months for an HIV blood test to read positive. It could take more than ten years for symptoms to develop, and a small percentage of HIV-positive patients remain asymptomatic indefinitely.

The danger with AIDS is that run-of-the-mill health problems become life threatening. T-cells fight obscure problems, like actinomycoses, which is a common fungus that rages out of control in the AIDS patient. Herpes can become herpes encephalitis. Toxoplasmosis, a parasite that causes a fleeting illness in a healthy person, can get into the

When HIV first cropped up in the 1970s, the medical community was mystified. Dr. Marvin Cooper, a hematologist I know, called me to ask, "Have you been hearing about a lot of Karposi Sarcoma in young men?" I told him that I had never seen one case in my career. It is traditionally an old man's cancer—not terribly aggressive, but something you get if you lived long enough and your immune system was weakened by your age. Suddenly, the instance of Karposi Sarcoma had skyrocketed in an inexplicably young and seemingly healthy community. This was the first red flag for me.

brain and cause dementia. So AIDS doesn't kill people, but the loss of T-cells and immunity makes the body vulnerable enough to succumb to a host of other problems.

We treat HIV with anti-retrovirals, which extend lives indefinitely. Anti-retrovirals are like a virus against the HIV virus—they infiltrate the viral cell (which is within a healthy cell) and corrupt its DNA. There are currently twenty-two different medications available.

The treatment scheme a physician assigns to a particular patient is called her protocol. The key to bear in mind while treating HIV is tailoring the protocol to the particular patient and constructing an appro-

The former surgeon general C. Everett Koop recommended that a new couple each get tested for HIV. If they were both negative, they could have sex using a condom and after six months if they were still monogamous, repeat the blood test. If it was again negative, they could assume that neither one of them was contagious with HIV, and they could commence unprotected sex.

sexually transmitted diseases

119

In the past twenty years, I've seen my best friend, caterer, two interior decorators, and my hair stylist all pass away from AIDS. They enriched my life, and I miss them dearly.

priate strategy. The days of complicated pharmaceutical cocktails for treating HIV are over. Usually, patients must take their medication once or twice a day at the most.

While the logistics are no longer complicated, these medications are very hard on the system in various ways. For example, some HIV medications cause diarrhea, so if the patient already has bad colitis, they have to try another kind of treatment. If you have a history of heart disease, you shouldn't take the medications that increase your risk of heart attacks. While in some lucky cases, physicians are seemingly able to control the disease, it remains very difficult to live with HIV. Regular doctor's visits become part of the HIV patient's life. It's like living with brittle diabetes.

It is very critical to take your medications when you have HIV. If you give the virus a chance to develop resistance, you become what AIDS specialists call a "treatment failure." Should this happen, "salvage therapy" is initiated, which is a much more aggressive and complicated attempt to reign in the virus.

While AIDS is the most dangerous of all STDs, it is luckily not that easy to catch. A very well-known, old story about a husband and wife illustrates this point. The wife became pregnant, and at the delivery, required a blood transfusion. This was before the days of testing blood for the virus. Seven years later, when she got pregnant again, HIV testing was mandated. It turned out she was HIV-positive, due to the blood transfusion she had received years previously. The babies and her husband, with whom she had had unprotected sex for seven years, were HIV-negative. This is no excuse for being irresponsible, but rather a reason not to be an alarmist.

PARASITIC

A parasite is a living creature that ranges in size from a one-cell organism (like amoeba) to a full-fledged bug (like lice). Like viruses, parasites by definition cannot live independently; they live off of a host creature. For example, a tic lives on a mammal—he must be attached to a warm-blooded creature so he can feed off the blood. Unlike viruses, parasites are not intercellular (i.e. they do not inhabit a healthy cell).

Doctors treat parasites in essentially two ways: we either ignore or eradicate them. We live in a symbiotic steady state with thousands of parasitic organisms at all times. The bacteria in our intestines are what make shit smell. We only bother to get rid of the parasites that bother or hurt us.

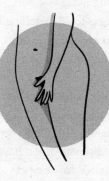

TRICHOMONAS

Trichomonas is a sexually transmitted parasite, though there are rare cases of women catching it in other ways such as at swimming pools. The parasite itself is a unicellular organism (like an amoeba) with a tail. An asymptomatic problem in men, trichomonas causes a greenish, foamy discharge and a burning sensation in women. Symptoms typically take about a week to develop after exposure.

Trichomonas is not in any way dangerous, but it is annoying, unpleasant, and best treated as soon as possible. We prescribe a topical or systemic antibiotic like Flagyl, which usually dispenses with the parasite in a matter of days.

LICE

There are two kinds of lice. Like herpes, one kind lives above the belly button, is relatively socially accepted, and is considered a minor inconvenience, usually for children. We call them head lice. The below-the-button lice are called pubic lice, and are more inconvenient, embarrassing, and harder to catch. Unlike herpes, the two kinds of lice seem to stick with their geographic zones; i.e. you can't catch pubic lice from someone with head lice giving you head.

As with other STDs, you can catch lice in nonromantic ways. An actress patient of mine caught lice from a costume that had been used by somebody else. Another patient went home to visit her family, and they insisted that her kid brother give up his bed for her. While he slumbered peacefully on the couch, she picked up some pubic lice to take back to New York with her.

The symptom of lice is terrible itching in the pubic area. Usually, we don't actually have to see the little bugs to diagnose the problem, but if you see something hopping around down there, it's a sure sign. If you really want tangible evidence, pluck a pubic hair—if you can find a small, glistening white dot attached, that's a louse egg.

There are many topical treatments we use for both kinds of lice. This usually involves a shampoo and fine-toothed comb to rid yourself of all the pesky eggs. Additionally, you have to clean everything that you've come in contact with for the previous two weeks, carefully removing all the eggs and dead lice.

* * * * *

MOTHER: "Is your generation worried about catching things?"

DAUGHTER: "Not really. Everyone I know is either in a long-term monogamous relationship, or doesn't really see much action."

MOTHER: "It seems polygamy is over. I almost never get patients like that anymore."

DAUGHTER: "Yup. It's like there's NO sex in this city."

MOTHER: "Aw. Have I ever told you about the sexual revolution?"

DAUGHTER: "Yup."

MOTHER: "After the pill but before herpes..."

DAUGHTER: "I've heard it before."

MOTHER: "There was like this incredible..."

Daughter: "That's enough."

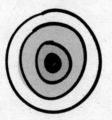

chapter eight

ABORTIONS

When I was twelve, I asked my parents if we could go to the pro-choice march in Washington D.C. They said, "Sure," figuring my interest would wane over the weeks leading up to it. On the morning of the march, I asked my Dad, "So are we going?" He was surprised that I remembered and cared, but we went to D.C. to participate in what was billed as the biggest march since the Vietnam antiwar protests. My most distinct memory of that day is of crowds of MEN on the side of the road with their pro-life literature. This is not to say that most pro-lifers are men, but that it's easy to be righteous about an issue that will never incontrovertibly affect your life.

This is the most opinionated chapter in this book, and I'm sure there are equally strong opinions across the chasm. A woman's right to an abortion is something I took to heart before it was even personally relevant, perhaps because it was part of my mother's practice and attitude. She and I agree; not every woman would elect to have an abortion, but no one should have such a personal and permanent choice made for her.

ABORTIONS—THE BASICS

An abortion is the termination of a pregnancy before the fetus is capable of independent life. Standard abortions occur between four and twelve weeks of pregnancy, but the procedure is legal in this country until twenty-four weeks of gestation. This number may seem arbitrary, but when *Roe v. Wade* was decided, no fetus had ever lived outside the uterus prior to twenty-four weeks of gestation. There have since been rare cases of babies who have survived with as little as twenty weeks of intrauterine development, most of whom sustained significant, permanent damage. The vast majority of abortions occur before the twelve-week mark.

Today in the United States we have two choices when it comes to abortions—medical or surgical. Surgical is the traditional method, where a physician dilates the cervix, evacuate the contents, and the patient goes home. Medical abortions require the patient to take a series of pills, which cause a spontaneous abortion or miscarriage. You may be more familiar with the medical abortion's unsnappy colloquial name—RU 486.

SURGICAL ABORTIONS

Standard surgical abortions involve gently dilating the cervix and sucking the contents out with a vacuumlike instrument. We call this a *suction curettage*. It generally takes about ten minutes, and depending on where you are, can involve local and/or general anesthetic.

First, the doctor performs a pelvic exam to establish the size and position of the uterus, both of which vary not only from person to person but from week to week of gestation. The physician then cleans the vagina with an antiseptic solution to reduce bacteria.

The first instrument used in an abortion is a tenaculum, which looks like tiny ice tongs. It holds the cervix in place—and sounds worse than it actually is. A steady cervix translates into less cervical trauma.

After the doctor has stabilized the cervix, she will begin dilation with what is unsurprisingly called a dilator. Dilators are gradated sticks that are used to gently open the cervix. The dilators are inserted in the cervical canal to stretch it and allow for the evacuation of the uterine contents. This is done gently and slowly. The idea is to avoid tearing the muscle or permanent trauma to the cervix.

The first and smallest dilator is about the diameter of the lead in a mechanical pencil, and the largest might be as big as your thumb. The

@vagina

I know that abortions can be embarrassing or even a big secret, but it is a very bad, dangerous idea to give false information when you are receiving medical treatment. The saddest cautionary tale I have about this dates from my residency. A woman came into the emergency room apparently having a miscarriage. Her pathology report came back, and it turned out this poor woman had uterine cancer. When we tried to alert her, we found that she had given us a false name.

desired cervical dilation is directly proportional to how pregnant the patient is. At six weeks, one dilates very little because there's a small amount of tissue and it's amorphous. At twelve weeks, there are more structures and tissue, so we generally dilate the cervix twice as much.

After expanding the cervix, the doctor passes a catheter (i.e. small hose) into the uterine cavity, which is attached to a suction apparatus. This removes the contents of the uterus. After this, a curette (i.e. a slim, curved, metal instrument) may be inserted to gently scrape the uterine walls to ensure all the tissue has been dislodged.

The patient is then brought into the recovery room, where she rests for about half an hour, and the medical team ensures there is no excessive bleeding or pain. After a surgical abortion, my instructions to the patient are, "Don't put anything or anyone in your vagina for two weeks." The cervix, usually closed tightly, is wide open after an abortion to any bacteria in the vagina. The primary activity of concern from a medical perspective is sex—potentially bacteria-carrying ejaculate shot right into the uterus is a very bad idea. Other ill-advised behaviors include douching, tampons, baths, and swimming.

Understanding that the vagina is already a relatively dirty place, abortion facilities and/or gynecologists will prescribe prophylactic (preventative) antibiotics postabortions for one to seven days. As with all antibiotics, you must finish all the pills or risk contracting a resistant

abortions

strain of infection. The infection rate for an abortion is about 2 to 3 percent, but you can cut that in half with antibiotics.

Two weeks after the abortion, the patient must return to her gynecologist for a checkup to make sure that she's not still pregnant and has no tenderness or sign of infection. This is also a great opportunity to discuss and evaluate the patient's contraceptive choices.

Complications

After your abortion, it is the doctor's responsibility to send all the products of conception (POC in medical circles) to a pathologist to identify placental tissue. If the pathologist doesn't find placental tissue, that means that the patient was 1) not pregnant; 2) she's still pregnant somewhere outside of the uterus, usually the fallopian tubes, i.e. an ectopic pregnancy; or 3) she's still pregnant in the uterus and the doctor missed it.

An untreated ectopic pregnancy can result in internal hemorrhaging, shock, or death. Extreme pain, dizziness, fainting, or abdominal distension could all be your first clue that this complication is happening to you. However, it's standard practice for the pathologist to call the physician in the absence of placental tissue, at which time the patient comes back into the doctor's office, repeats the pregnancy test, and has a sonogram. Sometimes, a sonogram is performed before the abortion to rule out the possibility of an ectopic pregnancy in the first place.

The incomplete abortion is another complication, meaning the physician failed to completely remove all the tissue in the uterus. This happens because doctors try to err on the gentle side, as the pregnant uterus is a soft, vulnerable organ. Should there be even a little fragment of placental tissue left behind, you will continue to bleed and your pregnancy test will remain positive. In that eventuality, you may have to be rescraped.

If the scraping is too vigorous, the complications can be more serious. As the physician scrapes the endometrium with a curette, she may accidentally and rarely perforate the wall of the uterus. The incidence of this depends on the skill of your doctor, the softness of your uterus, and

The Risks of Reproducing (or Not)

....

At any pro-life convention, they will either directly or indirectly mention an abortion fatality rate. While it is true that death is a complication of abortion, *you are one-tenth as likely to die from an abortion as you are from a full-term pregnancy*. Nothing about reproduction is risk free, but, in fact, it's very hard to die having an abortion. It takes a conspiracy of incompetence on the part of the patient, doctor, and staff. That said, celibacy is the only utterly safe option, but history and experience have shown that this is a very difficult, if not impossible choice.

....

dumb luck—regardless, this only occurs in less than 1 percent of cases. The appropriate course of action depends on the size of the hole, its location, and when during the procedure it happened. Treatment strategies range from basically nothing to reparative surgery.

A very rough abortion with vigorous curetting can lead to scarring of the uterine wall. Occasionally, the walls of the uterus can adhere to one another, ceasing menstruation. If you have an abortion, and do not have a period within four to six weeks, see your gynecologist. This problem can be treated, but, as with all else, the sooner diagnosed, the better. Postabortion infections, rare though they are, can also cause uterine scarring. A very small percentage of women will scar after a perfectly normal abortion. If left untreated, uterine scarring can lead to infertility.

Cervical stenosis, a condition where the cervix refuses to dilate, can be congenital, but is also associated with multiple cervical procedures (i.e. abortions). In the worst cases, the cervix is completely closed so that no menstrual blood can pass. If it's partially blocked, you'll still menstruate. Therefore, this condition is rarely diagnosed before labor. Cervical stenosis occurs in less than 1 percent of the pregnant population, but does necessitate a caesarian section. If you've had three or more surgical abortions, this is a potential risk.

abortions

129

On the flip side, cervical incompetence is also associated with multiple cervical procedures though it is typically congenital. Should your cervix prove incompetent, it would be unable to hold a pregnancy in the uterus. Physicians usually pick up this problem at about sixteen weeks of pregnancy due to the length and thickness of the cervix. Doctors treat this rather simply with a wide gauze suture (stitch or, in medical speak, a cerclage) on your cervix to keep it from dilating, allowing the patient a normal pregnancy sans jogging. Without the stitch, these women are relegated to strict bed rest.

THE MEDICAL ABORTION (RU 486)

Medical abortions are hormonal treatments that cause miscarriages, commonly referred to as RU 486 and known in the United States as Mifeprostine (brand name Mifiprex). Methyltrexate is another medical option; these days, it's not as commonly prescribed for abortions, but since it's used in chemotherapy, may prove easier to find. *These medications can be prescribed by any medical doctor*, but are only available to women within the first seven weeks of pregnancy, according to FDA guidelines. There's no tinkering with or dilating of the cervix, and no

---

Blood, Sweat, and Tears

One of the reasons I chose gynecology was that women make better, sturdier patients than men. This sometimes gets me into trouble, however, when it comes to postsurgical complications. How do you tell if, in the wake of an abortion, you are suffering a complication? "Blood, sweat, and tears," is a useful phrase I stole from an older gynecologist. If you are bleeding, if you have a fever, and if you're crying in pain, something may be wrong, and you have a responsibility to let someone know. It's embarrassing to show up in an emergency room with vaginal bleeding. Or you may not want to disturb your doctor, and I'm very happy that I have considerate patients. But if you get really sick, I'll be much less happy than I would have been if you had woken me up.

vaginas

scraping of the uterus. While there are several required trips to the doctor's office, most of the event happens in private, at home.

RU 486 consists of two medications; an antiprogesterone followed by a prostaglandin. Progesterone is the hormone of pregnancy—it promotes blood supply, food, and oxygen to the uterus. So if you diminish or oppose progesterone's affect on the uterus, the tissue that is meant to support a pregnancy will die, essentially killing the fetus. The major advantage of RU 486 is that it kills the tissue inside the uterus and in the fallopian tubes, so ectopic pregnancies are also eliminated.

Once the pregnancy is no longer viable, you still have to remove the contents of the uterus. The second part of medical abortions is a prostaglandin. You may recall that prostaglandins cause menstrual cramps as the uterus contracts (page 16). If you take them after terminating a pregnancy, they will help expel the contents of your uterus, much like a miniature labor.

This may sound like a simple two-pill process, but the FDA mandates certain procedures that make it less convenient. As RU 486 is only approved for the first seven weeks of pregnancy, most doctors will first perform a sonogram to ensure that you are no further along. Regardless, you have to go to the doctor's office to take your first pill, the antiprogesterone, in front of your doctor. Two days later, you must return for a sonogram or examination, as it's possible that your body has already naturally evacuated your uterus. If the pregnancy is gone, you don't need the second pill—the prostaglandin. If your uterus still contains extraneous tissue, you take the prostaglandin, and wait an hour in the doctor's office to make sure you don't throw it up. Then you go home, and that week you will have a miscarriage at home. This can be crampy and unpleasant, like an especially bad period.

This excessively cautious protocol may be simplified as physicians develop experience and confidence with the drug.

Complications

While they are certainly less intrusive, medical abortions have their own set of issues. Approximately 2 to 5 percent of medical abortions fail. In that case, you either repeat the whole process, or have a suction curettage. The FDA suggests medical abortions should only be done in a medical environment that includes a physician who can perform a surgical abortion in the event of a complication. So your general practitioner might be able to give you RU 486, but she should have someone local on hand who performs surgical abortions. This can complicate matters for rural women.

MEDICAL VS. SURGICAL

As with most things in gynecology, the choice between medical and surgical abortions comes down to very personal, subjective criteria. On the one hand, with RU 486 there is no surgery, anesthesia, and no instruments are involved. It's more private and therefore many women prefer it. If you happen to live in a pro-life area, you may not want to beat through a hostile picket line to have an abortion. However, it is a process that can be unpredictable, painful, and lonely. For some women, waiting for a quiet miscarriage, sometimes at home alone, is physically and emotionally stressful.

Surgical abortions, on the other hand, require a lengthy doctor's appointment, and then they are behind you. You will have a follow-up visit, but in the interim you can rest assured that you are no longer pregnant. Furthermore, you can be sure that, barring any complications, your discomfort will steadily decrease as the abortion recedes into the past. Additionally, because medical terminations have a failure rate, many patients reason, "Let me do it the old fashioned way and make sure it's done."

A SHORT, SUBJECTIVE HISTORY OF
ABORTION PRACTICES IN NEW YORK CITY

When I was a first-year resident in New York in 1969, abortions were still illegal. This left women to scrounge around for other, unpalatable options. We've all heard about the famous wire-hanger method, which

Classist Politicking?

There will always be abortions for women who can afford it. In the sixties, Park Avenue doctors would squirt a little blood into their rich patients' vaginas, and then they would rendezvous at the hospital, where these women would report inexplicable vaginal hemorrhaging. They were given safe, sterile abortions by their own physicians at an exorbitant cost and through complex logistics that were simply impossible for the vast majority of women.

involves passing a wire hanger through the cervix, hopefully stimulating uterine contractions, bleeding, and miscarriage. Unfortunately, the wire hanger not infrequently perforated the uterus, was not sterile, or occasioned upon a vital organ. But there were other horrendous and life-threatening trials women went through. Patients would douche with ivory soap, which could get into their blood stream and cause kidney failure. There were mysterious pills sold in bodegas, one was called Humphreys 11, that were rumored to be abortifacients (i.e. cause abortions). There was a caustic potassium permanganate pill that women would put in their vagina where it would burn through the skin. They'd bleed, and think they had started to commence an abortion when all they had were a holes in their vaginas. One woman took quinine, which she believed to be an abortifacient. All it did was make her nauseous and vomit. We admitted her for nausea of pregnancy and tried to make her better, while she was sneaking into the bathroom taking more quinine.

Imagine how complicated it was to treat women who came into the hospital after a botched, illegal abortion. Often, we were begging them for information so that we could save their uteri. Meanwhile, they were telling us deadpan that they had "fallen in the bathtub," "slipped on a broom," or "fell ice skating." The abortionists had their "patients" terrified that they would go to jail if they talked.

Abortion Story #1

I had a patient who, before I met her, became pregnant and had to have an abortion. A friend of hers gave her a phone number. When she called, they gave her specific instructions and an hour later she was at the mall, carrying a book with a red rose folded into it. At the curb, a black car pulled up, the door opened, and she got in. Imagine the terror of getting into a car, alone, with strangers. They took her out to the country where she was given an abortion on a kitchen table and immediately put back in the car, which took her straight to the shopping mall. She says it was the worst experience of her life.

Meanwhile, the only way to legally perform an abortion at the hospital was when the health (physical and mental) of the mother was impaired. Today it might sound ridiculous, but we tried to convince women who wanted abortions that they were suicidal because of their unplanned pregnancy. Of course, we couldn't let them in on the loophole, so you can imagine how difficult it was to convince these women that they wanted to kill themselves. They'd say, "NO, I'm not depressed, I just want an abortion." When it worked, this at least enabled us to do some abortions in a sterile and safe environment.

Family Lore

One of my great aunts once confided in me the story of her abortion when she was a married woman with three small children, aged two, three, and four, back in the 1930s. Every woman in the neighborhood knew the abortionist's number, because, according to my aunt, almost all of her neighbors—married women, with children—had had at least one abortion. He would come to the home and perform the procedure on the kitchen table. My aunt was sick for weeks afterwards.

Somebody called an ambulance and the paramedics found an unconscious girl on a bed in an empty room. At the hospital, the resident did a routine pelvic exam, and inadvertently reached through the giant hole in her uterus into her abdominal cavity, where he felt her liver. Her uterus had practically been torn in half, and could not be saved. She was so sick that when we performed abdominal surgery to save her life, she needed no anesthesia. Even three days later, when we took out the tube that helped her breathe, she remained nonresponsive. I was examining her hours later when she first opened her eyes. After this extraordinarily traumatic ordeal, her first words were, "Is the baby out yet?"

Safe, sterile abortions were the overwhelming exception to the rule. At night, the resident would admit anywhere from ten to twenty women who had clearly suffered at the hands of an inexperienced or unlucky abortionist. Most of the procedures I saw that year were incomplete, meaning that the pregnancy was no longer viable, but tissue was left in the uterus. This frequently caused sepsis, which is an overwhelming infection that leads to shock and death, if untreated. We gave these women massive doses of several simultaneous intravenous antibiotics.

As a resident, my job was to admit the patients and get them ready for the operating room, one of which was reserved for the droves of incomplete abortions. There were approximately twenty each day, of which there were always two or three very sick young women. Since we were ignorant about what had been done, what instruments had been used, and what kind of infection was involved, many of these women got hysterectomies. Many had kidney damage, adhesions, scarring, or abdominal pain that could last indefinitely. And ultimately, I would estimate that I saw about half a dozen young girls die from criminal abortions.

On July 1st of 1970, abortions became legal in New York City, and the TV crews came from all over. It was an exciting day. Overnight, admissions for incomplete abortions went from twenty each day to two or three a week. New York City abortionists made millions of dollars that year. They had toll free numbers advertised across the country. There were limousine services that picked patients up at the airport and brought them straight to the clinic. They flew in from Europe and Bermuda. There were whole hospitals dedicated to pregnancy termination. It was the gold rush for New York City gynecologists. I missed it.

PRESENT POLITICS AND THE
PARTIAL BIRTH CONTROVERSY

In the United States, it is legal to have an abortion up to twenty-four weeks of pregnancy. Should you choose to have an abortion after the twelve-week mark, it is considered a second trimester abortion. You may be more familiar with the catchy, political phrase "late-term abortion," though this is not a medical term.

There are two approaches to this: dilatation and extraction and induction. A dilatation and extraction is a more involved suction curettage, where the cervix is dilated and the contents are removed manually. Sometimes, the physician must collapse the baby's skull for an easier delivery—a procedure that is appalling to see, do, or experience. Apparently, this has just become illegal.

In an induction, the patient is admitted and the doctor attempts to get her into labor. Up until twenty-four weeks of pregnancy, the uterus

Mom's Manifesto
. . . .
Never underestimate the drive or desperation of a woman who cannot or will not be pregnant. The wards will fill up again with women falling in the bathtub and girls will die. Making abortions illegal does not stop abortions; it just makes abortions illegal.
. . . .

A patient was having a passionate affair with a married man, and she got pregnant. She couldn't have the baby, couldn't have it, couldn't have it! So we made the appointment for the termination. That morning, I stopped at the local deli and showed up with my iced coffee. When I got there, she was crying already. She sobbed, "I can't go through with it." I split my iced coffee with her and we had a chat. I said, "We've got a week ahead of us. Go home and think about it." The next week I showed up with an iced coffee, and again she was crying, "I can't go through with it!" So we split the iced coffee and had another heart-to-heart. The next week I showed up with two iced coffees and said, "I'm spending a lot on cab fare here, and we're not getting anywhere. If we do this every week for nine months, you're gonna have a baby." She decided to have the baby. Her son is now in high school, and she married the father. She's still a patient and I think very happy. The important thing to remember here is that nobody is pro-abortion; we are pro-choice. When you want a baby, we'll do everything we can to help you. If you don't want a baby for any number of good reasons, we'll take care of it for you. No one should have a baby they don't want, and no one should terminate a pregnancy they do want.

is understandably resistant to attempts at inducing contractions. Typically, it can take several days of medication (like prostaglandins, which cause fever and dehydration), with some risks, like a ruptured uterus, to accomplish your goal.

So even though the dilatation and extraction is an emotionally unacceptable procedure, it carries a far lower complication rate and is less traumatic to the patient, who remains asleep. Furthermore, women who go the less palatable route are in and out of the hospital, while women who must induce to terminate are usually on a delivery floor sharing rooms with women having full-term healthy babies.

Pro-life advocates and right wing politicians will have you believe that abortion is legal in this country up until the moment of birth. This is not true. After twenty-four weeks, medical efforts are made to save both patients—the mother and child. If at some point it is considered dangerous for the mother and/or baby to proceed with the pregnancy, she will be induced. However, the doctor must adhere to the safest medical course of action for both patients.

There are many reasons why a woman would elect to go through the difficult experience of a second trimester abortion. Amniocentesis results come in at about eighteen weeks of pregnancy, and sadly sometimes reveal chromosomal or genetic abnormalities. There are women who learn that their baby has massive anatomical problems, which may be incompatible with life. Sometimes there's no heartbeat. There are very young women who are so inexperienced, poor, or undereducated, they don't realize that they're pregnant until five months have passed or they have no means to readily acquire an abortion (the majority of counties in the United States have no abortion facilities). These are generally the most needy and desperate cases, but in most of these instances, there is good reason to terminate.

Second trimester abortions are much more difficult procedures than standard abortions, so therefore all of the complications of a first-trimester abortion are multiplied. Infection, perforation, incompletion, lacerations to the cervix or the uterine wall, and death are all nearer possibilities (remembering that the complications of full-term pregnancy always outnumber those of even second trimester abortions). There are very few doctors who regularly do second trimester abortions, and a lot of them are retiring. Should you find yourself in this unfortunate situation, your choices will be limited to regional medical centers for a dilatation extraction (depending on legalities), or an induction.

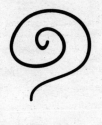

* * * * *

MOTHER: "Can I get political now?"

DAUGHTER: "How much more political do you want to get?"

MOTHER: "Women have been aborting pregnancy since the beginning of time...."

DAUGHTER: "I think it's already very clear how we feel."

MOTHER: "...never underestimate the drive and..."

DAUGHTER: "Mom. I heard you. Everyone will get it."

MOTHER: "...determination of a woman..."

DAUGHTER: "I'm leaving now."

chapter nine

REPRODUCTION

People will ask me what it was like writing this book with my mother. It was fantastic, educational, a great bonding experience, excruciatingly frustrating, and a hundred other things. Of course there were a few uncomfortable moments (I didn't really need to know anything about my parents' sex life, even if it was twenty-eight years ago), and we have pushed the envelope on what daughters commonly share with their moms. But I think it's important for all mothers to tell their children about their experiences bringing them into the world. Hearing about the extreme inconveniences, myriad sacrifices, nail-biting sessions, and profound discomfort, well, I'm just so grateful. Especially since my birth happened before epidurals.

They're not called reproductive organs for nothing. The main and original use of all the items we've been discussing is, of course, procreation. Here we'll hit all the high points, but pregnancy is intricate and unique to every woman. The tests and complications we discuss are just the tip of a huge iceberg.

SO YOU WANT TO HAVE A BABY

If you're ready and excited to get pregnant, there are a few timing and health issues to consider. Assuming that you are under thirty-five, and have had a relatively normal gynecological history, you should aim to have unprotected sex just before you ovulate. Recall that a woman ovulates fourteen days before the first day of her next period.

So if you have a twenty-six day cycle, you're ovulating on day twelve (counting from the first day of your period). If you have a thirty-day cycle, you're ovulating on day sixteen. Have lots of sex on and around those days.

There are a handful of general health considerations that, if relevant, would probably occur to a patient before she came to my office. If you are on any medication that is considered dangerous to pregnancy (e.g. Accutane) or if you have any kind of major illness that would make pregnancy more problematic, think long and hard about your decision after a thoughtful discussion with all of your physicians. If there is a family history of significant genetic disorders (e.g. hemophilia) or any genetic metabolic disease in the family (cystic fibrosis), consider genetic counseling.

WHAT KIND OF COUNSELING?

While to many, genetic counseling sounds like something out a science fiction movie, it's an increasingly common step for couples considering procreation. First, a geneticist or trained counselor takes a "pedigree," charting both families for diseases and potential genetic problems. The more you know about your family's medical history, the more accurate an assessment your counselor can make with regard to the risks your offspring may face. They are likely to recommend blood tests, which would reveal significant problems that might affect the baby.

Things they're looking for could be as manageable as diabetes, or as life-altering as cystic fibrosis. One in twenty people are carriers of cystic fibrosis, meaning that they have one recessive gene. Should you and your partner both have this recessive gene, the chances of your child having it are one in four. There are many recessive disorders that are linked to ethnicity and race. Tay-Sachs, for example, is the most serious of nine detectable genetic disorders that prevail almost exclusively in the European Jewish population, and leads to death within the first few years of a child's life.

BACK TO THE BABY

Assuming that you don't opt for genetic counseling and you are perfectly healthy, I urge you to consider a preconception consultation with your future obstetrician. She will recommend a host of things to prime you for pregnancy. Here's a sampler:

* Take folic acid. This is a critical vitamin for the development of the brain and spinal chord of the baby. You should be getting at least four hundred units of folic acid a day.

* Avoid unpasteurized cheese, a breeding ground of the bacteria Listeria. This causes a bad infection that seems mysteriously attracted to pregnant women and is a major cause of life-threatening infection and/or brain damage to the newborn.

* Eat meat well done to avoid toxoplasmosis—a parasite that is not threatening to a healthy person, but if you have it when you're pregnant, it could cause brain damage to the fetus. Wash your hands after handling raw meat and also avoid gardening and changing the kitty litter, because the parasite lives in cat feces.

* There are certain fish to avoid due to mercury levels. This information might change, but currently, the no-no fish include tile, mackerel, swordfish, shark, and probably tuna. The Environmental Protection Agency also cautions against eating fish you catch yourself, as waters close to shore tend to be more polluted.

* There are infections that you and your doctor have to be aware of—herpes, bacterial vaginosis, and Group B streptococcus are all associated with increased risks to pregnancy.

* Consider what medications you are on and if they are expendable. I've had patients on lithium who were too unstable to discontinue

medication and still wanted to get pregnant. But women who have a minimal emotional disturbance and are medicated might want to consider waiting until they are not on medication to undergo pregnancy, which is a tremendous emotional roller-coaster. Should you cease taking psychotropic agents for pregnancy, therapy is a good if not necessary alternative.

* * * * *

DAUGHTER: "So, Mom, if I came into your office, a healthy, twenty-eight-year-old, what would you say to me?"

MOTHER: "You are about to have the most fun of your life. You don't need contraception, and you have no reason to think that there's a fertility problem. Go home and have sex in every room of your house. Have sex at every time of day. Don't miss this opportunity for a sensual, glorious experience. Forget schedules, forget timing; there is no reason to make this anything but pleasant, romantic, sexy, and fun."

* * * * *

WHAT'S THE RUSH?

Age seems to be an ongoing issue in female reproduction and, unfortunately, medicine can't answer all of the toughest questions—especially the answers you might want. You are the most fertile in your twenties, and, for many of my patients, that's just not the best decade to become a mom. At thirty-five, you are 10 percent less fertile than you were at your most fertile. At forty, you're 50 percent less fertile. And at forty-five, the rate of spontaneous (unaided) conception runs at about 1 to 2 percent, and miscarriage rates skyrocket.

@vaginas

According to a *New York Times* article of March, 2004, Harvard Medical School has recently discovered evidence of continuing egg production after birth, which flies in the face of a major tenet of gynecology. Maybe we're not born with all the eggs we'll ever have. It is possible that this is the beginning of a new era in female reproduction and general health; wouldn't it be wonderful if we could trash the biological clock and stop arguing about HRT.

If you are over twenty-five, and you've made a lifetime commitment to the man of your dreams, you both want children, and you're economically ready, what are you waiting for? If you start early, and there are fertility issues, you've got some time to figure it out. Patients come in every year and ask, "How much time do I have?" My answer is always, "I don't know! You have less time than you had last year." It may happen that one day you'll be forty, blink your eyes, and say, "I forgot to have the babies." On the other hand, if you are thirty-eight, single, and are not prepared to have a child alone, get over it. You might find Mr. Right at thirty-nine, and it's never too late to have a baby; but it can become expensive, inconvenient, and not exactly biologically yours (i.e. you might need an egg donor).

I had a married patient in her late thirties who had always planned on having children. I said, "You're running out of time," and the instant that came up, her husband became impotent. They spent two years working that out in therapy, then they tried for a year or two and couldn't get pregnant. Then they did IVF (see page 161) for a year or two and they didn't get pregnant. Ultimately they needed an egg donor, because by the time they had even thought about trying, they didn't have the necessary extra few years to deal with potential hurdles. Fortunately, they have a beautiful baby now, but they got lucky.

HOW TO KNOW IF YOU'RE PREGNANT

The physical symptoms of early pregnancy are nausea, headache, urinary frequency, bloating, menstrual-type cramps, mood changes, libido changes, slight low back pain, and overwhelming exhaustion. The cervix gets softer and turns a little bluer when you're pregnant due to increased blood flow and congestion. But these are all pretty vague. The best way to tell if you are pregnant is to take a pregnancy test.

At-home urine tests are well over 95 percent accurate from approximately ten days after conception, or by the first day of your missed period. *Consumer Reports* is a great, current resource for grading at-home pregnancy tests for accuracy and ease of use. These tests measure the level of human chorionic gonadotrophic (HCG) in your urine. It is a pass/fail test as HCG is made by placental tissue—no other cell or organ makes this hormone. The major failing of the at-home pregnancy test is an occasional false positive result. Sometimes, if you are very irregular and your ovulation is late (i.e. you ovulate the day you do the urine test), there could be a cross reaction with the luteinizing hormone (LH—see page 13) surge, giving you a false positive. Urine can also be a teeny bit inaccurate due to dilution—if you drink six liters of water, the HCG may be so diluted the test comes back negative. It is a good idea, therefore, to use the urine from your morning pee. When in doubt, take the test again.

A blood pregnancy test is infallible, and unlike urine, quantitative. In a healthy pregnancy, HCG will double every two to three days. This is sometimes the only way to evaluate an early pregnancy for women

A Story That Made Mom Cry

I had a childless patient in her forties who mentored a young boy on weekends. I watched the relationship grow until one year she announced that she was adopting him. He called her "Mom" and there she was: a mother. Reproduction and motherhood are two very different things. One is a biological knack. The other is a true art.

In the 1960s pregnancy tests were a little more involved. A physician would inject a rat with the patient's urine, and then perform an autopsy on the rat. They would look at the rat's ovaries and if they were red or swollen, the physician concluded the woman was pregnant. Don't worry, PETA, this is seriously outdated.

who have had problems (e.g. miscarriages, difficulty conceiving, or prior problems in pregnancy) before.

THE TRIMESTERS

First Trimester

The first trimester starts with the first day of the last menstrual period and continues for twelve weeks. This is the period of organogenesis, meaning that starting with one cell (a fertilized egg is one cell, not two), the chromosomes fuse into the beginning of a whole new person. By the twelfth week, there's a recognizable human fetus approximately ten centimeters long.

In the first trimester, you should see your doctor every week until you establish that there is a viable pregnancy in the uterus. The doctor will monitor a host of other things (below) including your weight; they're looking for a three to five pound gain in the first trimester.

Major Tests

In your first trimester, physicians perform a lot of tests, because they want to anticipate any problems before they surface. A battery of blood tests will itemize overall health—physicians call this a complete blood count (CBC). An example of a red flag at this point is a very low platelet count. Platelets are a major player in blood clotting, and it would be extremely inconvenient and dangerous to find that out that the future mom has low platelets in a delivery room when she's bleed-

reproduction

147

ing excessively. Also, if the doctor sees that the patient is anemic, she knows to proactively address it. Over the course of pregnancy, fetuses demand iron to make their own red blood cells, possibly causing their moms to become anemic. There are many issues that could be catastrophic if not addressed, like syphilis. And there are things the hospital should be informed of at delivery, like if the patient has a certain blood type (e.g. RH negative).

This is also the time for a vaginal culture, to detect bacteria that could be harmful to the baby and should be eradicated by antibiotics. The doctor will do a Pap smear, to check for abnormal cells that could be dangerous as the cervix expands with pregnancy. She should also look for herpes, which is not necessarily dangerous but essential for the medical team to be aware of. And this is also the time to consider genetic testing (see page 142).

At five weeks, there is a sonogram to rule out an ectopic pregnancy, which is when the fetus is growing somewhere other than the uterus, usually in a fallopian tube. One to two percent of pregnancies are ectopic, which, if allowed to progress, will grow until the tube ruptures. These pregnancies are extremely dangerous—a ruptured ectopic can cause a fatal hemhorrage. Conversely, an unruptured ectopic can be treated fairly easily. At six or seven weeks, there's another sonogram to look for the flicker of a heartbeat. Ten percent of fetuses do not have one and are therefore not viable. In medicine, this is called a missed abortion, and the physician empties the uterus with a D&C (page 227) so the patient can try again.

Risks

The first trimester is the most tenuous stage of pregnancy. Things that happen in the first trimester can be catastrophic, while the same incidents swould not be a big deal in the third trimester. For instance, if you catch German Measles at eight weeks, it can cause brain damage and cataracts in the fetus. If you catch German Measles the day before you go into labor, maybe the baby will be born with treatable German Measles.

∙∙∙

A patient came in for a routine visit and was surprised to learn she was pregnant. To her horror, she had been at a club the prior weekend and taken some pills that a stranger gave her. She asked me, "What do you think?" and I said, "How can I tell you?" She had a healthy baby, but that was eight months of unnecessary worry.

∙∙∙

There are three major areas of concern in the first trimester:
1. Medication
2. Radiation
3. Infection

Medication

There are both legal and illegal medications to consider. As soon as you start thinking about getting pregnant, absolutely discontinue all illegal drugs—pregnancy, especially first trimester pregnancy, is not the time to do a line of coke, smoke a joint, or shoot heroin. Recreational drugs are associated with their own set of problems, a major component of which is total ignorance about what exactly you're taking, smoking, or snorting. In pregnancy, these issues multiply, and while some women may get through pregnancy while doing drugs, there are few things sadder in medicine than an addicted newborn.

Legal drugs include social and therapeutic drugs. Social drugs are caffeine, cigarettes, and alcohol. Nobody who has a tenth of an ounce of brain tissue should be smoking cigarettes, period. But when pregnant, it's even stupider because it effects the oxygen the mom's body absorbs, thereby diminishing oxygen to the baby. Cigarette smoking does not cause birth defects, but low birth weight.

* * * * *

reproduction

149

DAUGHTER: "Even though you smoked half a pack of cigarettes a day."

MOTHER: "Ten cigarettes."

DAUGHTER: "I'm not even runty."

MOTHER: "I compensated with food."

* * * * *

Alcohol is associated with a syndrome called *fetal alcohol syndrome*, which causes a neurological deficit and dysmorphic (funny shaped) face. Alcohol is an absolute no-no for the first trimester.

Limit your consumption of caffeine to two helpings each day. This includes coffee, tea, cola, certain nuts, coffee-flavored ice cream, and candies. If you overdo caffeine, it constricts your blood vessels, potentially limiting blood flow to the baby. Less seriously, a baby born with a caffeine addiction is no fun—think about how irritable it makes a real caffeine addict to give up coffee. Does anyone want to give a newborn another reason to cry?

Therapeutic medications are nonprescription drugs that we all take for a host of ailments. Avoid these as much as possible. For instance, instead of Nyquil, try old-school remedies like eucalyptus, menthol, or a nice steam bath. Stay away from herbal treatments—they may have their own set of undocumented risks. Don't take anything you don't know everything about.

Times Change

In the fifties, I knew a doctor who would tell his patients, "Don't quit smoking now, it'll make you too anxious." *He* was anxious, as were most doctors in the fifties, about having to do a cesarean section, which was at the time a risky and complicated procedure. The smaller the baby, the less likely that would happen.

Radiation

Radiation is linked to miscarriages and structural birth defects, though there is very little way for the medical community to gauge exactly what the risks and results are. We are all exposed to radiation in computer monitors, televisions, and on airplanes, so it's a good idea for your first trimester to stay at least a few feet away from monitors and televisions. You may want to limit air travel.

The most obvious source of radiation is an X ray. You'd be amazed how many X rays you get in the emergency room that could be avoided if you tell them you might be pregnant. Dental X rays are okay—they're far from the uterus and a negligible amount of radiation. However, why go if you can wait until at least the second trimester?

Infection

If you are sick, the rule of pregnancy is to treat the sickness, but include the obstetrician in the decision making. Let's say you have pneumonia and don't take antibiotics because you don't want to hurt the baby; your being sick certainly isn't good for the unborn child and

X Rays and Pregnancy

A patient of mine was told as a teenager that she would never get pregnant, which is a horrible, unfounded thing to say to a young girl. On her honeymoon she was in a car accident. In the emergency room, she had multiple X rays of her pelvis to evaluate her injuries because she told the physician that she couldn't possibly get pregnant. A week later she realized that she was late for her period and was indeed pregnant. She went to a geneticist who attempted to calculate the radiation, who ultimately had to admit that he just couldn't tell her what her risks were. This was so devastating, it destroyed her marriage. If you are having unprotected sex and wind up in the emergency room, tell your physician you might be pregnant even if you think it's highly unlikely.

if you die, that kid's prospects aren't too good either. It is unfortunate that most significant illnesses increase the risk of miscarriage. It's untimely to get sick while pregnant, but the chances of avoiding any potential pitfalls are good if appropriate therapeutic choices are made.

Miscarriages

From the moment you learn that you are pregnant up to your twelfth week, your chances of having a miscarriage are as high as 50 percent. From the first day of your missed period, to the first sonogram where we see a gestational sac (at about five weeks), the chances of miscarriage go from 50 to 25 percent. Two weeks later, when we do another sonogram and see a heartbeat, it drops to under a 10 percent risk. And at twelve weeks, with an apparently healthy fetus (i.e. with a heartbeat), your risk of miscarriage drops below 1 percent.

An abnormal but not necessarily terrible sign in the first trimester is vaginal bleeding. This is what we call a "threatened abortion," because your body is threatening to miscarry. Fifty percent of the time vaginal bleeding is the harbinger of a miscarriage. Most of these miscarriages happen because the fetus is genetically abnormal—the pregnancy was just not meant to be. For the remaining 50 percent, the pregnancy continues perfectly normally. Should you commence vaginal bleeding in your first trimester, usually your doctor will see you, do a sonogram, and if there is still a healthy pregnancy, advise bed rest.

There are sadly many ways to miscarry. A spontaneous complete abortion is a miscarriage in which you bleed and pass the tissue. A missed abortion is when the heart stops beating and you don't bleed, meaning the pregnancy has died or lost viability but it stays in the

Medical Speak

There is no such thing as a miscarriage in medical terminology. Whether you choose it or not, physicians call an early end to pregnancy an abortion.

Bed rest may or may not have scientific validity. Lying down, there's no gravitational effect of the pregnancy pressing on the cervix. If you're bleeding vaginally, the blood can stimulate contractions. Being prone helps. When resting, there's maximum blood flow to the uterus, because the mom isn't using that much. Ultimately, regardless of whether bed rest works or doesn't work, it enables you to say, "I did the best I could." If you end up having a miscarriage, right or not, you will scrutinize the choices you made and want to know "why." So many patients point at something they did and blame themselves. It's important to take all the steps you can to help the pregnancy.

uterus. As stated in the abortion chapter (see page 125), there are medical (RU 486) and surgical options for treating this. Typically, the choice will be yours, but occasionally the physician will strongly recommend one or the other (e.g. if you're hemorrhaging, we don't have time for you to take a pill and wait). An incomplete abortion is a miscarriage in which not all of the tissue is expelled and there are still some fragments of placenta left behind, causing you to continue bleeding. This usually requires a dilatation and curettage (D&C) or some mechanical method of emptying the uterus. A blighted ovum is a miscarriage in which the gestational sac forms inside the uterus but no embryo develops. These are detected when the uterus fails to grow, the placental hormone levels stop going up at an appropriate rate, or there's no embryo or heartbeat seen when there should be.

These days most miscarriages are diagnosed before pain and bleeding. It's no less sad and tragic, but rushing to the hospital in the middle of the night with vaginal bleeding is thankfully rare.

reproduction

Second Trimester

During the second trimester, from the end of the twelfth week to the end of the twenty-fourth week, the fetus grows from four to twenty inches, and weighs approximately one to one-and-a-half pounds. The primary mandate after the twelfth week is nutrition. Adequate weight gain is ten to fifteen pounds in the second trimester.

This is the March of Dimes diet for every day of your pregnancy, but especially from the second trimester on:

* One quart of milk or its equivalent
* Eight ounces of protein
* Four slices of bread or the equivalent
* Two servings of leafy greens
* One yellow serving (apple, banana, potato, etc.)
* One source of vitamin C (orange juice, grapefruits, etc.)
* Eight glasses of water

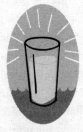

The second trimester is probably the most pleasant, least risky point of your pregnancy. You should see your doctor about once a month for blood pressure, urine, and weight checks. At this point, the uterus is very resistant to contractions. Miscarriage rates run at less than 0.4 to 0.6 percent. The nausea is better, but the patient isn't so big that she's uncomfortable. This is a good time to take a vacation.

Tests

The major test of the second trimester, though not performed all the time, is the amniocentesis. At about seventeen weeks, an obstetrician draws a small amount of amniotic fluid (from the gestational sac within which the baby comfortably floats) with a long needle. The amniotic fluid, membranes, placenta, baby, and umbilical cord are all fetal in origin—they are all cut from the same cloth. So the liquid drawn in an amniocentesis can tell you a lot about the genetic makeup of the future child, i.e. if the cells in the amniotic fluid have a normal chromosome count, then the baby does as well. Usually, the obstetrician will do a sonogram and an amnio concurrently, and between the two diagnostic tests, the physician is able to diagnose a host of chromosomal and structural problems.

Any chromosomal abnormality is bad news. However, some are less bad than others; some may be incompatible with life, while others are not a cause for concern. For example, the geneticist might find an

Chromosomal Abnormalities 101

Almost every human cell (except the red blood cell) has forty-six chromosomes in it— that's twenty-two sets of autosomal (i.e. nongender related) chromosomes and one set of sex chromosomes. Forty-six chromosomes with two XX chromosomes is a girl, forty-six chromosomes with one X and one Y is boy. Forty-five and forty-seven are bad numbers when it comes to chromosomes. There is not one documented case of increased intellectual performance associated with an abnormal chromosome count, and the names and complexities of these conditions are too many to list here. The most common chromosomal abnormality is when there is an extra chromosome at the twenty-first pair. This adds up to forty-seven chromosomes over all, as there are three twenty-first level chromosomes where there should only be two. In medicine, we call that trisomy 21 but you're probably more familiar with the condition as Down's syndrome.

reproduction

155

abnormal chromosome in the amniotic fluid that he has never seen before. The next step is to test the parents; if one of them carries the same chromosome and enjoys a normal life, then the baby is almost surely fine. I've seen this a half-a-dozen times, and some fanciful geneticists postulate these may be the beginning of a new chromosomal dynasty.

For a twenty-five year old mother, the risk of a chromosomal abnormality is less than 1 in 1,000. At thirty-five, it is approximately 1 in 250. At fifty, if you are one of those rare people lucky enough to get pregnant, the risk of a chromosomal abnormality is 1 in 10.

So not every woman should have an amnio. The test carries a 1 in 250 risk of miscarriage, infection, or ruptured membranes. At thirty-five, the risk of a chromosomal abnormality is about the same. So when the risk of the test is greater than the risk of what you are testing for, the American College of Obstetrics and Gynecology (ACOG) recommends you do not routinely do the test. Of course, there are exceptions to this (e.g. if you have a history of chromosomal abnormalities in your family), but generally we start recommending amnios when the patient is thirty-five.

If you choose not to have an amnio, but are over thirty-five or desire a chromosomal analysis, there is another test called Chorionic Villus Sampling (CVS). This is where an obstetrician extracts a small fragment of the placenta with a needle under sonographic guidance. The advantage of the test is that it can be done earlier in the pregnancy (at about ten weeks) and is faster, preventing the necessity of a later abortion should you find something abnormal. CVS unfortunately carries a higher complication rate than an amnio—a 2 to 3 percent increase in the rate of miscarriage.

Sonograms remain very important because structural abnormalities are far more common than chromosomal irregularities. Again structural defects can be profoundly significant or not such a big deal. A profoundly significant problem, for example, is a baby who lacks kidneys (called Potter's syndrome)—there is no way for this child to live. An extra pinky, however, is not such a big deal.

... is a very good thing, as long as you are enjoying a normal pregnancy with no high risk factors and your doctor hasn't instructed you to abstain. The penis keeps the vagina elastic and lubricated, making pelvic examinations much less uncomfortable. The ejaculate contains prostaglandin compounds (see page 16), which will make the.uterus contract and soften the cervix.

Approximately 4 percent of babies in this country are born with structural birth defects. Fifty percent of these babies suffer no ill effects—a birthmark, for example. The remaining 2 percent of all births have significant congenital defects that require surgery, medical care, or further days in the hospital.

The other major test at around seventeen weeks is called an alpha feto protein. This is a protein that's very high in the fetus. If there's a hole or a defect somewhere in the baby, this protein can leak out into the amniotic fluid, cross the placenta and circulate in your body. An elevated alpha fetal protein can signal a very significant birth defect.

Third Trimester

The third trimester is a month longer than the other two, spanning from the end of the twenty-fourth week to delivery at the end of the fortieth week. This is when obstetrics dominates the picture—is the baby growing enough? Is the mother's blood pressure normal? Is the mother diabetic? Is she dilating prematurely? Is she having too many contractions too soon? Is the baby in a good position?

While over the first twenty weeks of pregnancy, the baby's size is pretty predictable, in the third trimester, weight dispersal is based on many factors, not all of which are understood. Girls are slightly lighter than boys. Nutrition is an important determinant, and then there's always pesky genetics. You should continue the pregnancy diet and gain ten to fifteen pounds.

The last ten weeks of pregnancy is a good time for prepared child-birth classes. Take a tour of the hospital where you're going to deliver. Go over the procedures and your thoughts about labor and delivery with your obstetrician. Start thinking about names.

Tests

At twenty-eight weeks your medical team will make sure you do not have diabetes through a simple blood test. They may do a sonogram between thirty-two and thirty-eight weeks to make sure the baby is growing adequately. And they will want to do a vaginal culture to look for group B strep, a bacteria that isn't good for a baby on the way through. If you have it, it's easily treated with antibiotics.

Complications

There are two diseases unique to the third trimester of pregnancy. Both of these ailments are essentially asymptomatic as they occur today, because physicians should pick them up way before the patient develops symptoms.

Pregnancy Induced Hypertension (AKA Pre-Eclampsia or Toxemia)

Blood pressure can become a very serious problem, and sometimes mandates hospital admission and early induction of labor. Pregnancy induced hypertension is characterized by generalized vaso-spasm (all the arteries in the body contract), creating a high-pressure environment. Should this happen, you might notice that you are very swollen as the pressure in the arteries squeezes water out of your blood and into the nearby tissue. The first thing your physician might look for is protein in your urine; the high pressure in the arteries forces protein out of the blood vessels and into the kidney, and hence into the urine. If you manage to sneak the first two symptoms past your doctor, or if your blood pressure climbs precipitously, the lack of blood flow to your brain could cause generalized seizures. But if you see your doctor regularly, she will hopefully notice your blood pressure go up before you exhibit any of the symptoms of pre-eclampsia.

Pre-eclampsia occurs more in younger patients and first-time pregnancies, and we just don't know why. There's a Nobel Prize waiting for the person who discovers the cause of toxemia. Some scientists think it's caused by a particular element of the patient's diet, while others believe a mysterious placental chemical causes blood pressure to shoot up. Research on this topic is ongoing, and lately more focused on the placenta as possible culprit.

If you have pre-eclampsia, you will be admitted to the hospital so they can try and control your blood pressure, evaluate fetal well-being, and deliver the baby if and when things turn sour. If toxemia sets in after thirty-six weeks of pregnancy, your obstetrician will almost definitely induce and deliver you. The more serious the pre-eclampsia, the earlier you want to deliver the baby, because if the mom is really sick, then the baby is in danger too. Doctors must always assess what will be better for the baby *and* the mother.

Gestational Diabetes

Pregnancy is a diabetogenic state, meaning that it stimulates latent diabetes because the placenta makes anti-insulin compounds that cause the mother's blood sugar to go up. When gestational diabetes is diagnosed, it means changing the mother's diet and possibly putting her on insulin until birth. The idea is to keep the mother's blood sugar as close to normal as possible so the baby can have a relatively normal level of sugar in her blood stream.

From a delivery perspective, the dangerous component of gestational diabetes is that diabetic babies are fat. This generally leads to a higher incidence of cesarean sections. Also, once born, the baby will need to be closely monitored to make sure their blood sugar is stable. In the first few days of their lives, the danger is that, since they are adjusted to a high-sugar environment, they will overproduce insulin resulting in dangerously low blood sugar.

Some more unfortunate news is that diabetes associated with pregnancy is frequently a harbinger. Up to 50 percent of women who have gestational diabetes will develop it in their later years.

AND THEN THERE'S THE BABY

There are tens of things that can go wrong on the baby's end of things, and while there are several hundred specifics, most of these issues fall into these major categories: abnormal position of the baby, abnormal placental function, abnormal growth of the baby, undesirable conditions of amniotic fluid, and undesirable conditions of the cervix among others. Look out for our next book.

INFERTILITY

At least 10 percent of all couples are infertile, meaning that out of all the male-female pairs that try to get pregnant, one in ten has a medically addressed roadblock. For women over thirty-five there's an additional 10 percent of infertility (meaning 80 percent of women between thirty-five and forty have no trouble conceiving). Out of the 20 percent that remain, at least 50 percent do nothing about it, and a quarter of them have readily addressable issues (e.g. they're having sex at the wrong time of the month or using lubrication that is actually spermicidal).

Bad Eggs

I had a patient once, I believe she had a Ph.D. in rocket science or something brainy, and she was having trouble getting pregnant. She was only thirty-two. I sent her to an infertility specialist who gave her a battery of tests, and told her, "You have bad eggs." She came storming into my office twenty minutes later and ranted, "I'm a rocket scientist! Don't talk down to me! I can understand whatever it is that's wrong with my eggs." So I called up the infertility guy as she blew steam out of her ears in my office and asked him to explain to me in medical terms what he meant by "bad eggs." And he said, "What? She's got bad eggs. They're bad. Not good. Bad." Today we call it "poor egg quality." The medical community certainly does not understand all the facets of reproduction, and we can't control most of them.

In Vitro Fertilization

In vitro fertilization (IVF) is when fertilization occurs outside of the body or in a test tube, as opposed to in vivo, which means "in the body." An infertility expert extracts the follicle through the vagina or abdomen with a big needle under ultrasonic guidance. Generally, the mother will be given drugs beforehand to make her "super ovulate," so the physician can retrieve more than one follicle (up to twenty or more). Meanwhile, the dad has to masturbate in a bathroom. The product of his and her experiences are put together in a test tube and hopefully fertilization takes place. The fertilized egg divides until it is at the stage where it would ordinarily be implanting in the uterine wall (approximately three to five days). Then the specialist redeposits the little tyke in the mother's uterus, hopefully to implant. In the best of circumstances, IVF only works 40 percent of the time, and that number shrinks as the mother gets older (if she's using her own egg). And, this whole thing is extraordinarily expensive (around $10,000 from start to finish per cycle).

Problems that cause infertility can be divided roughly into thirds. About 30 percent of the time, the problem is the "male factor" (low sperm or poor sperm), another 30 percent of the time the problem is the female reproductive structure (blocked tubes, inhospitable cervical mucus), and another 30 percent of the time, the problem, ladies, is the egg. A host of less common problems accounts for another 10 percent: e.g. thyroid imbalances, sperm allergies, pituitary malfunctions, and inadequate mucus, to name but a few.

Of these previously infertile couples who manage to conceive, up to 50 percent of the pregnancies end in miscarriage. About half of these are called "chemical pregnancies" meaning the woman was a few days late with her period, technically pregnant, and then menstruates. It seems just like a late period when it's actually a miscarriage.

Another 25 percent of the formerly infertile couples that achieve pregnancy are "clinically" pregnant. They're two weeks late with their period. They have all the symptoms of pregnancy, and a sonogram will show a small sac in their uterus. And then the sac doesn't grow, or there was a little teeny blip of a heartbeat on the sonogram and suddenly there's no heartbeat. These are early losses, usually between five and twelve weeks gestation.

It helps to remember that the human reproductive system is remarkably complex—every time it works, it's a small miracle. In a system of such intricacy, a high rate of loss is, on a rational level, understandable. There are a huge number of things that can go wrong in conception and pregnancy, resulting in what we insensitively term in obstetrics, "fetal wastage."

* * * * *

MOTHER: "You didn't happen until the second cycle."

DAUGHTER: "Don't sound so accusatory."

MOTHER: "I lost my mind. It is so easy to fall into a horrible imaginary black hole of infertility. It's discussed on every TV show, it's in every magazine. The minute the cycle goes by and you're not successful, it's depressing and anxiety provoking. People start telling you terrifying, sensational infertility stories."

DAUGHTER: "But Mom, it was just the second month. What were you so crazed about?"

MOTHER: "That I didn't get pregnant the first month."

DAUGHTER: "And we wonder why I'm so impatient."

MOTHER: "In retrospect, I wish it had taken a little longer."

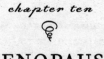

chapter ten

MENOPAUSE

The one thing that Mom won't tell you about her menopause is how great she looks. I mean, she really looks at least ten years younger than she actually is. Good genes are (thankfully!) part of the picture here, but she credits hormone replacement therapy (HRT), a youthful attitude and assorted well-packaged face creams. While it may not be for everyone, and research on this explosive topic continues, it seems that HRT can be an important component of looking and feeling fabulous. This is just my opinion, built on close observation of Mom for the past twenty-eight years. Boy, does she look great.

Menopause literally means last period, and typically occurs in a woman's late forties to early fifties. It's impossible to know when your last period is going to be, so menopause is something retrospective. You look back and say, "I haven't had a period in about a year so." And that was that.

MECHANICS OF MENOPAUSE

Remember, we're born with a finite number of follicles and that's all we'll ever have (for a hopeful caveat, see page 145). The follicle consists of an egg surrounded by cells that make estrogen and progesterone. So when we run out of follicles, we have no more eggs, can no longer reproduce, and we cease to make any appreciable amounts of sex steroids.

The best news is one stops menstruating—no more pads, tampons, cramps, PMS, etc. The bad news is that most women will

Only three female animals we know of have a menopause. They are all large mammals that live past fifty years of age. Care to guess who?*

experience a host of unpleasant symptoms, which are her body's response to a lack of estrogen. A lucky 20 percent of women experience very mild symptoms, while approximately another 60 percent complain of the most common symptoms, such as hot flashes (for specifics, see page 168) for six months to six years. For an unlucky 20 percent, menopausal symptoms can continue indefinitely.

WHY MENOPAUSE?

It's been estimated that women live up to 30 percent of their lives postmenopausally. This doesn't really make a whole lot of sense in terms of the reproductive goals of most species. Women spend about one-third of their lives sterile, while men are reproductively capable until the day they die, churning out sperm from puberty to the grave, in some cases.

On the one hand, we could think of this as an accident of evolution. We evolved into bodies that could expect to be around for thirty years, and, within that period, we would never run out of follicles. If this is, in fact, an accident of evolution, then we should replace those hormones when we stop making them, much as we would replace the thyroid or the adrenal gland if they stopped functioning. However, there are those who argue that menopause is a natural transition in the life of the human female. When looking back at evolution, they might

* Elephants, humpback whales, and human females are the only creatures who go through the "change of life."

●●●

I had a thirty-one-year-old patient come in recently because she had-
n't had a period in three months. The poor woman had premature ovarian failure—essentially, an early menopause that can strike someone
as young as thirty. This is an unexpected catastrophe, both because
the woman is sterile and because of the health implications of
menopause (see page 168). There seems to be a familial element here,
so it is definitely worth asking your mom when she had her menopause.

DAUGHTER: "Mom?"
MOTHER: "I was forty-nine."

●●●

suggest menopause is a useful marker for a new stage in our female
predecessors' lives; the sign that they have become "grandmothers"
who take care of the young and allow the younger generation to go
hunting and foraging. On the one hand, menopause is a unique event,
unparalleled in the course of human biology. And in other ways it's just
like all the other stuff we outlive—our eyesight, our thyroid, our
joints, and a hundred other things.

We may never know which of these theories is "right," but there
are undeniable life changes after the ovaries die and most of them
aren't terribly pleasant, or worse, are life threatening. For good or ill,
estrogen and progesterone are our sex hormones. They are the hormones that make us female. They make us *us*. And to deny ourselves
that hormone when we stop making it because of fear, because of studies that are flawed in their population selection, because of medical
trendiness, and because of a host of variables we cannot control may be
a rash decision. See the section on Hormone Replacement Therapy
(page 171).

PERIMENOPAUSE

It's very popular today to talk about the perimenopause or the "time around the menopause." The most common definition of perimenopause is the time period "within five years of your last menstrual period." For 60 percent of women, there are no warning signs; they have no symptoms before the cessation of menstruation.

In approximately 20 percent of women, estrogen levels drift down as they approach menopause. They will occasionally skip a period or bleed less. The hormone change may also trigger menopausal symptoms (see page 168), even though there's still some menstrual activity. It's like being caught in between two worlds. This is classic perimenopause.

If you think this information might apply, your gynecologist can test your hormone levels, assessing estrogen or follicle stimulating hormone (FSH). The pituitary may produce more FSH as it attempts to stimulate a dead ovary. So a high FSH (over fifty milliunits per milliliter) or low estrogen (under twenty picograms per millileter) is defined as menopause. Women with these hormone levels will not usually menstruate, though they may still have a burst of estrogen significant enough to get the uterus to respond with a menstrual period.

Another unfortunate 20 percent of perimenopausal women will have a stormy menopause, not because their body is not making enough estrogen, but because it's making too much. Much as a diabetic will frequently overproduce insulin and become hypoglycemic before they develop diabetes, an older woman's body may try to make more

Hypochondria, Anyone?

One morning I woke up sweating. This went on for a good week before I decided that I needed HIV and tuberculosis tests and maybe a chest X-ray. One of the young nurses in my office whispered, "Could it be the menopause?" and I looked at her, deeply offended, and said, "I'm not old enough! I'm only . . ."

The time leading up to menopause can present a confusing picture, for patient and doctor alike. There are some symptoms that can mask themselves to appear innocuously consistent with this stage of life. But, if your periods last more than twice as long as normal, if your cycle is consistently less than twenty-one days from first day to first day, or if you're spotting between periods, these can be signs that there's something wrong. Don't allow yourself to be blown off if you have these symptoms, because endometrial cancer is more easily missed in a perimenopausal woman than in a postmenopausal woman. When a postmenopausal woman has some spotting, doctors pay attention and search for a problem, but for perimenopausal women, unusual bleeding means nothing most of the time. You or your physician might assume that these symptoms are all just part of the "changes," but stamp your feet and show them this sidebar.

hormones to compensate for the impending death of the ovaries. These women will spot and/or get heavier more frequent periods, and fibroids, if they have them, will grow in response to the estrogen. Breasts can also become more sensitive.

The standard of care right now for a difficult perimenopause is a low-dose birth control pill. This suppresses ovarian estrogen production, evening out the waves of hormonal events that can naturally make for a rocky transition.

The difference between the birth control pill and hormone replacement therapy (a common but currently controversial treatment for menopausal symptoms, see page 171) is that the birth control pill is stronger because it's suppressive. The hormones need to enter the system with enough potency to convince the patient's ovary not to work. Once a woman is menopausal and there is no period, there's also no estrogen so a much lower dosage of hormones is still effective.

The most common menopausal symptoms include hot flashes, night sweats, sleep disturbances, and a compromised sex life. Hot flashes are a sudden flush of body heat that often lead to profuse sweating and discomfort. They can last from thirty seconds to a couple of minutes—it's a flash. Night sweats are just like hot flashes, except that they happen in the middle of the night. Patients report that these are more intense and longer, but it could just seem that way because they happen at 3 A.M. Night sweats may be a contributing factor to sleep disturbances, but many women report insomnia unrelated to sweating.

Then there's sexual dysfunction as a corollary to menopause. While sex drive naturally diminishes with increasing age, it can be challenging to continue having sex after menopause. Without estrogen maintaining a healthy vagina, it becomes dry and fragile. The vagina is lined with squamous epithelium (like all of our skin) that is fifteen to twenty cells thick or more. It's elastic, it stretches, and it's moist. The squamous epithelium in our vagina is extremely sensitive to estrogen stimulation. In the hormone's absence, that thick squamous epithelium can narrow down to one or two cells thick. There is no moisture. The elasticity disappears. Without estrogen, the vagina atrophies, making sex somewhat painful or in some unfortunate instances, impossible.

The labia and the mons, all of which are estrogen-dependent, also start to lose their characteristics. Pubic hair grows sparser until nearly vanishing. The labia become thin and can virtually disappear so that the external genitalia resembles a prepubertal girl's.

Other symptoms of menopause that are harder to pin on the event itself are mood changes and depression. These could just be part of growing older, but they are generally improved by hormone replacement therapy (see page 171).

Osteoperosis

Bone is living tissue, much like coral in the ocean. There are cells that make bone (osteoblasts), and there are cells that destroy bone (osteoclasts). It's a constant turnover of bone eaters, followed by bone

Almost every cell in the human body has a receptor site for estrogen. These are like locks for which estrogen is the key. When these receptor sites are stimulated, meaning they are plugged with estrogen or a substitute, that cell responds by either becoming more metabolically active, dividing or becoming healthier. These receptor sites are everywhere. For example, there are plenty of receptor sites in the brain. In tests where they gave MRIs to animals on estrogen, they saw the brain getting healthier, bigger, and more active. There are receptor sites in the skin, and when given estrogen, we can see the skin become thicker, moister, and more elastic. There are estrogen receptor sites in the vagina, which is the most dramatic organ in terms of estrogen sensitivity, and without the hormone, the vagina atrophies; blood vessels disappear, the walls thin, and moisture is a thing of the past.

builders, followed by eaters, followed by builders. When the bone eaters and the bone builders are in equilibrium, we have great bones. But without estrogen, the bone builders slow down, so that the bone eaters begin to overwhelm the system. This leads to thinner bones, a condition most commonly known as osteoperosis.

Bone loss is its most dramatic in the six years after the last period. This is not just an inconvenience. Depending on a number of variables, osteoperosis can leave a victim bedridden for the rest of her life. Even for those relatively mobile osteoperotics, fractures become much more likely, and over 20 percent of women will die within one year of breaking a hip. Less dramatically, there are those who have chronic pain from fractures, and those who have increasingly stooped postures.

Calcium and exercise are essential, period. But for women past menopause, they are no longer optional, regardless of their HRT decision, because these noncontroversial choices stimulate healthy bone production. However, hormone replacement therapy (see page 171) is

menopause

169

There are all sorts of situations that can cause a body to start losing bone, though in situations other than menopause, this problem will generally reverse itself. For example, whenever a woman's body is put into an estrogen-deficient state, bone loss occurs. Eating disorders can cause a woman to cease menstruation, and therefore estrogen production. So a sixteen-year-old girl can sustain osteoperosis if she has a bad enough eating disorder. It may seem ironic, but women who cease menstruation due to hyperathleticism can suffer the same result. Certain medications, like diuretics, thyroid replacement hormones, and steroids, can cause bone loss as well. Women who are breast feeding will lose bone because all their calcium is going into the milk, and they're usually not menstruating either. But in all these situations, there are generally healthy, estrogen-producing years to regain the bone that was lost. Menopause is trickier.

the only treatment strategy that prevents bone loss almost completely, by directly stimulating the osteoblasts (bone builders).

There are medications besides estrogen to help maintain healthy bones. There are biphosphonates like Fosomax or Actonel, which slow down the bone eaters (osteoclasts). These medications bring your bone renewal rate to a new and slower equilibrium and are generally suggested once there has already been some bone loss. Estrogen prevents it from happening in the first place.

SERMs (selective estrogen receptor modulators) are another option. These estrogen look-alikes help prevent bone loss and breast cancer. The most famous SERM is called Tamoxifen, a medication primarily used to treat breast cancer. Raloxifen (brand name Evista) is a different SERM, which is used to treat osteoperosis.

TREATMENT STRATEGIES

NOT HRT!

For those of you who do not want to take systemic hormones (synthetic hormones that circulate via the blood) there are few options for you to treat your menopausal symptoms. Of course, a healthy diet, plenty of sleep, low stress levels, and exercise are always a good idea, though their affect on menopausal symptoms is undocumented.

With regard to sexual function, you must adopt a "use it or lose it" strategy, meaning you have to keep having sex in order to be able to continue having sex. Six months without penetration could lead to a narrowing of the vagina that would make penetration uncomfortable or even impossible. If a woman will consider the use of hormones for treating her menopause, there's a vaginal ring called Estring that releases small doses of estrogen over a three-month period. And there's a low dose estrogen pill that women can put in their postmenopausal vaginas (brandname Vagifem). These treatments will only help the vagina, and not alleviate any other symptoms (i.e. you'll still get hot flashes).

HORMONE REPLACEMENT THERAPY (HRT)

HRT is pretty much what it sounds like—it's replacing the post-menopausal woman's missing sex hormones with synthetic ones. *This is the only scientifically proven method of treating menopausal symptoms and associated medical issues.* Some women take it for a few months, others for the rest of their lives. If you live in a remote arctic outpost, you may not be aware that HRT is one of the most raging debates in women's health, with reasonable arguments on both sides.

HRT is very similar to the birth control pill. Most women on HRT are taking both estrogen and progesterone. If you've been reading carefully, then you might be wondering, "Why does the post-menopausal woman have to take progesterone?" It's true that estrogen will cure almost all (99 percent) of women's vaginal dryness, and almost always cure their additional symptoms. However, estrogen

The original, classic synthetic estrogen is conjugated equine estrogens, brand name Premarin. This compound is extracted from reproducing female horses' piss—i.e. PREgnantMAres'uRINe.

without progesterone (AKA unopposed estrogen) can overstimulate the lining of the uterus and cause endometrial cancer. Progesterone prevents this from happening. For women who have had hysterectomies, however, estrogen alone is fine.

Estrogen comes in pills, as a patch, and as a ring that stays in your vagina for three months, just like systemic hormonal birth control (see page 70). The most common progesterone used up until now has been medroxyprogesterone, brand name Provera, which only comes as a pill.

Annoying Side Effects of HRT

Going on HRT can invite all the symptoms of premenstrual syndrome back into your life. Breast pain is especially reported among HRT adherents, as is a ten to fifteen pound weight gain. On some courses of treatment, women get their periods back and resume a life similar to that before "the change."

What's Everyone Making Such a Fuss About?

It seems that the two big problems with estrogen therapy are breast cancer and cardiovascular events.

Breast Cancer

It's not that estrogen stimulates a perfectly healthy, normal breast cell to mutate into cancer. The hypothesis is that the estrogen may stimulate a cancer to grow that otherwise might have not. The risk is extremely small, in my opinion, but there may be an increased risk when taking HRT.

There is a reduction in breast cancer *mortality*, however, for women who get cancer when they're on estrogen therapy. In other words, you might be slightly more likely to get breast cancer (we're talking a difference of a fraction of a percent) but you have a dramatic reduction in the risk of it killing you.

There are many ways of looking at statistics and breast cancer. Ninety percent of women who get breast cancer have never been on hormone therapy, not even for a day. Furthermore, if estrogen played the primary role in causing breast cancer, there would be a plateau in the incidence of breast cancer after menopause, because there is no estrogen in a postmenopausal woman. But the incidence keeps increasing throughout a woman's life into her eighties.

If you have an extraordinary family history of breast cancer, as in your twin sister, your mother, and all three aunts had breast cancer, you should be under a specialist's surveillance and estrogen therapy may not be for you. However, if you are at low risk for breast cancer and you are lousy with menopausal symptoms, hormone therapy might be a good choice.

Cardiovascular Events

The second area of concern with HRT is cardiovascular. The early work on estrogen therapy showed a dramatic improvement in cholesterol, reduction in heart attacks, strokes, and arterial diseases of all kinds. Estrogen replacement was thought to prevent heart disease. However, the original study that demonstrated these benefits was flawed in that it was self-selective. The women who chose estrogen might have been more health conscious, prone to exercise, and a low-fat diet. These women were all immediately postmenopausal and when they started with the estrogen they were relatively young. This group was followed for many years with dramatically good results.

After this study was published, when women had heart attacks, their cardiologists would say, "Of course you had a heart attack, you're not on estrogen." Well-meaning physicians would put these women on estrogen, unknowingly causing them to become *more* likely to have a second heart attack than women who were not put on estrogen. At least we learned early on that estrogen doesn't help if you already have heart disease. In fact, if you have coronary heart disease, going on estrogen could make your condition worse.

But Wasn't There Some Other Controversy?

The biggest study of HRT, called the Women's Health Initiative (WHI), came out in the summer of 2002. This study leveled a surprising blow to the HRT movement by citing an increased risk of breast cancer and vascular events when postmenopausal women were given estrogen and progesterone HRT.

While the study was certainly large (with thirty thousand female volunteer subjects) and blind (i.e. the women were not told which group they were in and they were all given identical pills), it was not flawless. The researchers ensured that virtually none of the volunteers had any menopausal symptoms. They knew if they chose women who were symptomatic, they might compromise the "blindness" of the test. Many of the women who were treating their stormy menopauses with HRT already did not want to risk giving up their hormones. Furthermore, the average age of the volunteers was sixty-four; i.e. many of them were *well* beyond their menopauses.

Half-way through the study the researchers realized that among the ten thousand women on Prempro (progesterone and estrogen), there were eight more breast cancers, six fewer colon cancers, three fewer hip fractures, and anywhere from ten to fifteen more vascular events (heart attacks and strokes) than in the placebo group. However, while the increase in health problems associated with Prempro approached statistical significance, it was actually *not* statistically significant.

The Premarin segment of the study was suspended in the spring of 2004 due to an increase in strokes. There were five more strokes than in the control population for an increased risk of 1 in 2000, which is not statistically significant. There were no increased risks of breast cancer or heart attacks, but they abandoned both the Prempro and Premarin studies early because it's unethical to continue giving people medication that may cause complications.

Anytime you consider a large study like this in making your own healthcare decisions, really scrutinize the numbers. When they say, "It doubles your risk of X," ask what your risk was to begin with. If it was 0.3 percent, and doubles all the way to 0.6 percent, it is still less than 1 percent. This kind of increase is significant when you're interested in statistics for an entire population, but when you're a unit of one, these numbers should not be terribly frightening. Think of it this way—how much colder are you when the temperature drops from five degrees to four?

What I Tell My Patients
Some women have no problem with the menopause. But if you are uncomfortable and miserable with menopausal symptoms and want hormone therapy, you should begin within three years of your last period because this does not show an increased cardiovascular risk. After ten years postmenopause, one has already developed some narrowing of the coronaries and a slight increase in arterial sclerosis. For these women, estrogen might be something that's moving the problem along or accentuating those cardiovascular events whereas in healthy coronaries, estrogen prevents problems. If you're healthy, estrogen helps to keep you healthy. If you're not healthy, it probably won't help you.

There is a real battle going on for the hearts and minds of women everywhere, and there are very strong lines within the medical community. The anti-estrogen people say that however well you feel on HRT, it's all in your mind. That it's all a big placebo effect. The pro-estrogen people say, "That's bullshit! You feel better, you think more clearly, and you have a better sense of well-being."

The anti-estrogen people say that whatever goes wrong can be addressed individually. If you have elevated cholesterol, take statin (Lipitor, Zocor, etc). If you have bad bones, take a biphosphonate (Fosamax or Actonel), or a SERM (Evista). If your skin is sagging, see a plastic surgeon. Some are trying psychotropic agents like Prozac and Zoloft to relieve night sweats, and they claim these treatment methods alleviate 50 percent of symptoms. Colonoscopies become routine after fifty, so the improvement of colon cancer on HRT is negligible. These people are looking at illness and disease. They're not looking at a woman and her life. Tackling menopausal symptoms piecemeal doesn't address a woman's day-to-day existence. Nothing helps the insomnia, the night sweats, the hot flashes all day, and the vaginal dryness (to name the most common menopausal ailments) like estrogen.

The pro-estrogen people feel it's good for your brain, skin, heart, bones, colon, vagina, attitude, sex life, and your chance of getting a good night's rest. And people who love it agree! I guess you can tell which side I fall on.

The estrogen controversy is ongoing and I'm not sure it will be solved in our lifetimes. Your decision should be predicated on a couple of things. First, it's not one study; it's an accumulation of studies. To recap, a lot of the negative studies have been based on giving estrogen to women who are many years postmenopausal. Ten years after your last period there have already been some changes in the body, so you are introducing a hormone to a different physical person than a woman who is less than a year from her last menstrual period. There are equally strong studies suggesting that women who start hormone treatments right after their menopause have few or no bad health repercussions.

Mom's Story
....

I've been on it now for ten years. I tried to reduce it, and I've actually forgotten it once or twice, and my night sweats and hot flashes come right back. So I may be one of those people who have hot flashes till the day I die. Both my parents had heart attacks and died when they were ten or fifteen years younger than I am right now. I am on Lipitor, and my current angiogram shows that my coronaries are wide open. I wish I could point to a better lifestyle or diet than my parents, but I don't get much exercise and I love butter. My personal example certainly doesn't carry the weight of a scientific study, but I credit estrogen for my improved cardiovascular health.

....

On the other hand, I can't say absolutely that it's good for you. If you're having a great menopause and you feel fabulous, then no one's telling you to go on hormone therapy just because it should be good for you. I'm saying that if you're miserable, don't suffer. Don't be frightened. Go on it for a year, and then try and discontinue if you're petrified. Try to go off it every couple of years until you don't care about hot flashes or you don't get hot flashes

A final thing to consider is that most medical professionals agree that the important thing about HRT is monitoring how long you have estrogen in your system. For instance, if you have a late menopause you may have an increased incidence of breast cancer because that's another ten years of estrogen stimulating your breast. It's not the source of estrogen, but the length of time that your body is exposed. Therefore, the reverse is true. If you have an early menopause, earlier than forty-five, consider hormone therapy *at least* until you get to the age of the average menopause (fifty-one).

* * * * *

DAUGHTER: "So we need a verbatim dialogue for the end."

MOTHER: "What's a verbatim dialogue?"

DAUGHTER: "You know, at the end of each chapter we have a

cute little exchange that I take from our discussions while writing the book."

MOTHER: "Oh, right."

DAUGHTER: "So we need one."

MOTHER: "How 'bout this one?"

DAUGHTER: "Alrighty then."

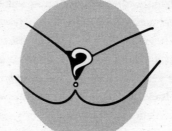

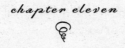

chapter eleven

THIRTEEN MYTHS OF GYNECOLOGY

Most of my friends should know better, but, on the whole, they've managed to come up with some of the most remarkably unenlightened gynecological questions and concerns out there. Which leads me to charitably conclude that they're not alone when they worry about a topical anomaly, thinking that their bikini wax–induced ingrown hair is some sort of obscure labial cancer. Or when they think burning when they urinate is a sure sign of some incurable, awful, tropical, fatal ailment they caught. In the Bahamas. Two years ago. It's okay, there are no such things as stupid questions, just silly women who didn't buy this book and will continue to worry about their wayward G–spot.

MYTH # 1: THE BUMP

You're taking a shower and find a bump somewhere in or around your genitalia that wasn't there before. Of course, it's cancer. You bang down your gynecologist's door first thing the next morning, haggard and panicked, eager for the first time ever to tear off your pants and reveal the fatal blemish.

Truth

Bumps are almost always just bumps—ingrown hairs, sebaceous cysts (a benign growth), pimples of all varieties, stuff like that. I once told my husband, "I need a medical term for a bump. Patients need something they can hang onto." Although he isn't a doctor, he came up with "topographical anomaly," and "dermatological aberration." Use those big words to explain to your boss why you're late for work.

The only bump worthy of concern is the wart. If it looks like a wart (a cauliflowerlike surface), or if your sexual partner mentions warts, you should see your gynecologist who will be happy to get rid of them for you. Genital warts are a relatively innocuous if unsightly strain of the human papilloma virus (HPV) and should be removed because they are contagious, terrifically unattractive, and can grow quite large. But bumps are not cancer. They're not even life threatening.

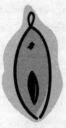

MYTH #2: VAGINAS ARE SMOOTH

It always seems to be in the middle of the night that women get courageous enough to investigate their bodies. Whereupon one might discover what seems like an irregularity, (e.g. a ridge, rashlike surface, uneven texture, cactus flower*) or several bunches of them in the vagina.

Truth
Bumps and ridges on the vaginal walls are normal. They are supposed to be irregularly shaped. There can even be little bumps on the cervix, called Nabothian cysts, which are perfectly harmless.

• •

*We're joking about the cactus flower. If you find one of those growing in your vagina, call your doctor.

MYTH #3: SECRETIONS ARE BAD

Any vaginal secretion is a sign of an infection.

Truth

Vaginal secretions are healthy and protective. The rule of thumb is if it doesn't itch, burn, or smell (much, much worse than usual), then it's normal.

MYTH #4: THE G-SPOT

There are women who claim there is an area in their vaginas that is highly sensitive and extraordinarily pleasurable. Many folks (especially in the adult entertainment industry) claim this patch, when stroked, rubbed, or stimulated, is THE destination event of any woman's sexual experience. Certain scientists have even claimed that in utero, this area grows into the G-spot on women and the prostate gland on men, lending a certain amount of evolutionary backing to an otherwise dubious and unprovable claim.

Truth

Tissue samples of the so-called G-spot area show absolutely no difference from the vaginal tissue next to it. There are no extra nerve endings or blood vessels. Certainly YOUR G-spot may be a very real, wonderful thing to you, and if so, that's fantastic for you. But you'll never find a shred of physical evidence.

Caveat

Just because science can't back up a claim, doesn't mean it doesn't factor into people's lives. People feel pleasure in all sorts of different ways, times, and places. The mind can convince the body of almost anything. Your cerebral cortex is your primary erogenous zone. But if you have never been able to locate that pesky G-spot, try somewhere else you never thought of, like the back of your knees or neck.

MYTH #5: YOU CAN LOSE SOMETHING IN YOUR VAGINA

It's the middle of the night, and you can't get your diaphragm/tampon/whatever out. You start sweating. Then a clammy chill comes over you. You're shaking you want it out so badly.

Truth

If your diaphragm, tampon, or pretty much anything nonporous stays in your vagina for an extra few hours, it's no big deal. It's not a passageway into the rest of your body, so you can't "lose" anything in there.

You can retrieve almost anything from your vagina if you're calm. Go for the rim of a diaphragm or the edge of a tampon. Try squatting. Seriously. Bear down (as if you were having a bowel movement) so that whatever's in there is pushed lower, closer to where you can reach it. Finally, if you're not shy, your boyfriend/husband sexual partner/roommate could remove the item for you, because they'll have a much better angle. If you're really in a bind, any emergency room or gynecologist can get it out for you.

MYTH # 6: THE VAGINAL ORGASM/FEMALE EJACULATION

There are women who claim to have orgasms during vaginal intercourse, without any clitoral stimulation. Then there's the more obscure, but still tall tale of female ejaculation, which involves some sort of fontlike expression of vaginal secretions in mimicry of the male money shot.

Truth

We thought we'd go for a double buzz kill on this one. Most scientists suspect that the "vaginal" orgasm is still a clitoral orgasm that happens when thrusting indirectly stimulates the clitoris. It's a nice, convenient, lazy-man's orgasm of choice, but it's just not that much of an option for most women. As for female ejaculation, we're not sure why anyone would choose to ejaculate, but there just aren't any organs that could make this actually happen in the female external genitalia. We're just not built that way.

Caveat (not a total buzz kill)

There are women who have had their clitorises removed, who have later been able to achieve orgasms (this is generally possible for women who had orgasms before they lost their clitorises). We don't know how they do it. There are also transsexuals who have artificial vaginas who claim to have orgasms with their new, synthetic genitalia. So don't let us rain on your parade.

MYTH #7: BREASTS AND LABIA ARE SYMMETRICAL

Many women come to me distressed over a breast that's much bigger than the other. When the rare patient ventures on a mirror-aided journey of self-discovery only to find that one side of her nether region is visibly larger than the other, she's understandably upset.

Truth

Usually, these women are making a mountain out of a molehill (chuckle), in that there just isn't a significant difference between right and left. Most women don't really notice the difference in breasts or labia, although perfectly symmetrical breasts are as rare as two identical grains of sand. Only occasionally is the difference dramatic (one A-cup and one C-cup breast, or one labia hanging below the other), and the only cure is plastic surgery.

We only *tend* towards symmetry. No human being is perfectly symmetrical; hands, feet, ears, breasts and labia are generally well-matched sets, but they're also unique.

MYTH #8: SEX IS ALL PLEASURE, ALL THE TIME

Many women feel that if sex is uncomfortable or painful, there must be something terribly wrong.

Truth

It's not uncommon for sex to be occasionally uncomfortable for a whole lot of reasons.

You Can Have Too Much of a Good Thing

Sometimes the mind is willing but the body isn't able. You've had sex seven times in twelve hours, and on the eighth go-round, your vagina may be dry and irritated. Goo is essential in this situation, or try getting out of the house.

Get Yourself a Copy of the Kama Sutra

If you're having vaginal intercourse in a position where the thrusting penis (or whatever) hits the cervix head-on with force, it can push your uterus, stretching all the ligaments that hold it. This can cause a charley horse sensation in your abdomen after sex or it can hurt when it's happening. Subtly change your position, angling a bit to either side of the cervix.

And Then There's Bum Luck

If you're having vaginal intercourse during ovulation, there's a big, juicy follicle at the surface of your ovary waiting to burst. If your partner hits that big, juicy follicle at just the right angle, he will rupture it. The offended ovary, our analog to testicles, will make you hit the ceiling in pain, because you kind of just got kicked in the balls. Now that's a phone call in the middle of the night that is certainly understandable, and I usually get them from the poor guy who thinks he did something terrible to you. If it's the middle of your cycle and you're not on the pill (which would stop you from ovulating) you probably just popped the ripe follicle. This pain subsides in three to four hours, but it hurts like hell and it's scary. Thankfully, this is very rare.

@vaginas

MYTH #9: MY OVARY HURTS / I CAN FEEL MYSELF OVULATE

Women frequently entertain the notion that they "know" when they're ovulating, that they feel ovarian pain, or that they can just sense when their ovaries are "in trouble." Patients have come into my office specifying "ovarian distress" on their medical history.

Truth

In general, patients should try to stay away from diagnosing themselves, and in specific, pain of the ovaries is not something you're really able to identify. Abdominal pain could signify a problem with your colon, bladder, abdominal wall, or a pinched nerve. No matter where it comes from, pain is a very vague, similar message to your brain, and sometimes, it can be misleading. As a side note, women who claim to know when they're ovulating are wrong 50 percent of the time. You may think your gynecologist is interested in these sort of projections, but she's not.

MYTH #10: THE MAGIC HYMEN

The first time a woman has sex, she expects there to be blood from a severed hymen.

Mom's History Corner

In medieval times, when a lord married, he would display a bloody sheet the morning after the wedding. Not only did this announce the purity of his new bride, but guaranteed that any offspring were sure to be his. This more likely indicated a lack of foreplay than virginity. And in any case, I find it hard to believe that there was that much blood and suspect that most of it was usually drawn from the chicken they served at the wedding dinner.

In the early nineties, I had a patient who asked to have her hymen sewn back together again. She was over thirty, a professional, and was going home to Afghanistan to marry the man her father had picked for her. She claimed she would be in terrible trouble and physical danger if she were not a virgin on her wedding night. So we threw some stitches in across the vaginal opening so there would be some bleeding and obstruction with vaginal intercourse. I don't know whether it was successful or not. She never came back.

Truth

Among women, a virgin is someone who hasn't had vaginal intercourse. Whether you bleed your first time or not is a matter of luck more than anything. Athletics and tampons also tend to impact relative discomfort and bleeding, so these days it's pretty common for virgins to have a bloodless first go-round.

MYTH #11: CLOTCHA!

There is something about a menstrual blood clot that inspires terror in most women. Those little brown clumps in the toilet, on their pad, or clinging to their tampon pack an emotional wallop.

Truth

Clotting is a good thing; it's a sign that you're not a hemophiliac. Unless you are taking medicine to thin your blood, outside of your arteries and veins, healthy blood will clot.

When your period is just starting, menstrual blood leaves the wall of the uterus and floats in the cavity, where it clots. There's an enzyme that dissolves the clot called plasmin. So what you see on your tampon is blood that's been clotted and dissolved.

@vaginas

The only downside is that women with clottier menstrual blood tend to have more painful periods, as the uterus has to contract more and the cervix may dilate to allow for solid material to pass. Women who have clottier periods have a low plasmin-to-menstrual blood ratio.

Caveat

Don't look at the clot, look at the overall volume of blood loss. If you think that you're bleeding 50 percent more than usual, and it lasts a full day or more, speak to your gynecologist about it.

MYTH #12: THE MYTH OF THE UNCLEAN

Many women think that their periods make them unclean, to the point where they should sexually abstain while they are bleeding. There are even religions that promulgate this theory.

Truth

Human beings are normally capable of sexual function 365 days out of the year if they so desire. If you abstain from sexual activity during your period, this may lead to increased sexual activity later in the cycle, which would make you more likely to conceive. This accomplishes a major goal of most religions—enrollment.

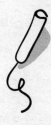

We're Fascinated by Prostitutes

Think about it—they don't take off for their period. They use cotton balls, wedging them up against their cervix, leaving plenty of room for business to proceed as usual.

MYTH # 13: MEDICINE CAN SOLVE ALL
THE MYSTERIES OF THE HUMAN BODY

Truth

Unfortunately, most of the time doctors don't really know why something bad happens to a patient's health. For most ailments, there are myriad possible causes, a large number of which are unknown. And even when she knows what's wrong, no physician is able to cure or even effectively treat every illness.

* * * * *

DAUGHTER: "What surprised you most about being a doctor?"

MOTHER: "That a huge percentage of my work is psychiatric. There's anxiety, depression, psychosomatic illnesses. There is a psychological component to almost every visit."

DAUGHTER: "When did you realize this?"

MOTHER: "My first year in practice, a patient came in doubled over in pain. I said, "How long have you had this pain?" and she said, "Since October seventeenth." I said, "What happened on October seventeenth?" She explained it had been her wedding day. When I suggested there was a connection, she screamed at me and stormed out. Maybe if I had said it a different way or waited...."

DAUGHTER: "What kind of training did you have in psychiatry?"

MOTHER: "Two weeks."

DAUGHTER: "You can't be too hard on yourself then."

@vaginas

MOTHER: "It's harder to say to a patient, 'See a therapist' than, 'You have cancer.'"

DAUGHTER: "How many times a year do you say to someone, 'You should consider therapy.'?"

MOTHER: "Every day. Well, I *think* it every day."

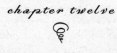

chapter twelve

SIGNIFICANT PROBLEMS OF THE OVARIES AND FALLOPIAN TUBES

My best friend Kaena goes to a warm and fuzzy new-agey doctor who uses words like "welcoming" and "beautiful" to describe the images of Kaena's reproductive organs. This is fine—Kaena and I are very different people. One day, Kaena went for her checkup and, suddenly, it seemed, her ovaries were no longer "lovely" or "perfect." She had endometriosis and it had taken root on her left ovary. For a woman who feels that her reason for being on this earth is to become a mother, this was a very hard thing to hear. Even though it's not serious or that unusual it can be fertility threatening. She tells me now that she's not sure what was worse, hearing about the endometriosis or having to go on the pill (again, we are very different). Ovaries can be beautiful, but they can also be little tyrants—kind of like the children they beget.

OVARIES

Almost all problems of the ovaries involve a growth of some kind, i.e. something you can see on an ultrasound or feel during a pelvic exam. There are hundreds of kinds of these growths, and luckily, the vast majority are not medically concerning. The toughest facet of ovarian care is distinguishing between things you should worry about and things that will go away on their own.

The Navy figured out that sending sound waves through water, then evaluating how those waves bounce back, is a pretty reliable method for determining what if anything is out there (e.g. a submarine). They refined the technology to the point of being able to outline submerged vessels with ultrasound, also known as a sonogram. Someone brilliant said, "Well, fetuses float in fluid, maybe we could see them too." And ultrasound was introduced into obstetrics as a means of evaluating intrauterine babies without subjecting them to any radiation. Now, sonograms are a standard diagnostic tool of gynecology, and essential in evaluating ovaries, because most ovarian problems evidence themselves with physical growths. Ultrasounds show us the surface of the ovaries and the consistency of any growth, which as you'll see (page 193) can be very important information.

FUNCTIONAL CYSTS

Recall that follicles (the hormone-producing egg packages) are also cysts, meaning that they are fluid-filled sacs. Once a month, one lucky cyst moves to the ovary's surface in a completely expected and essential part of human reproduction and hormone production. All of the cells in these cysts are normal. Sometimes, these completely mundane cysts misbehave in some way, and generally that's when they get our attention.

Functional cysts include perfectly normal follicles, generally picked up towards ovulation on the surface of the ovary as an incidental finding during a sonogram. Normal cysts doing abnormal things are also termed functional cysts, and these can be alarming for the patient, but generally not so for the doctor. These cysts are a by-product of female human reproduction, i.e. they are a direct result of ovulation. They rarely grow large enough to threaten healthy ovarian tissue, and they never spread or invade other nearby organs—99.9 percent of the time, these cysts will go away on their own.

Sonograms—Two Choices

There are two kinds of sonograms used to evaluate the pelvic organs. An abdominal sonogram is done on your lower tummy, while a vaginal sonogram is done you-know-where. The vaginal apparatus looks like a big vibrator, and when the technician puts a condom on it, you too will find this comparison hard to ignore. This approach, as aesthetically displeasing as it might be, gives you a much closer, clearer picture of all the pelvic organs.

The complexity of functional cysts from the physician's point of view is making an absolutely certain diagnosis. The first question doctors ask of the ovarian cyst is, "Is it simple?" By this, we mean are the walls of the growth smooth and the contents clear. We also make sure

Ultrasounds—Don't Forget Them

Should your gynecologist recommend a follow-up sonogram to evaluate an ovarian cyst, DO NOT FLAKE OUT. This can mean the difference between a long, healthy life and a rapid, fatal decline. My florist's wife came in to see me, and I felt a mass in her pelvis. We did a sonogram, it looked abnormal, and one week later I operated on her and removed the early stages of ovarian cancer. Five years later, she is still healthy and well, and her oncologist will soon return her to my care. I had another patient who happens to be a nurse. When we found a slightly abnormal-looking cyst on her ovary, I recommended a follow-up sonogram. She blew me off, and in the course of that year got four sonograms from four different doctors, all of whom became increasingly concerned. When I saw her again a year later, she had advanced ovarian cancer and needed a hysterectomy. Her prognosis is not as optimistic as it could have been. Sonograms do not hurt, they do not take a long time, and they are absolutely essential in gynecological healthcare.

there's a normal amount of blood going to the cyst. A bumpy surface or increased blood flow are both signs of a more serious problem. Physicians answer these questions with an ultrasound.

Additionally, doctors look at the bigger picture. If the patient is postmenopausal and it's been more than five years since her last period, then any ovarian growth is very concerning. Ostensibly, this woman is no longer ovulating, so her ovaries should be nice and quiet. Within a woman's fertile years, the ultrasound is more important in shedding some light on the situation. If, for a menstruating woman, the cyst looks normal at the time of her first ultrasound, her physician would probably recommend a "wait and see" approach, which basically means a follow-up ultrasound within one menstrual cycle. Usually, the cyst will simply disappear, and that would be the end of it. If the cyst is still in the same place, and is growing, then the patient and her physician need to start considering next steps.

Types of Functional Cysts

Persistent Functional Cysts
Sometimes a follicle or several follicles will refuse to rupture, and instead, stay on the perimeter of the ovary—producing hormones. These are called persistent functional cysts and result in three conditions: one, an above normal level of estrogen in one's system; two, no eggs to make babies because the follicles tend not to release them; and three, it delays menstruation because the continuing hormones prevent the lining of the uterus from shedding.

Often women who experience this suspect they might be pregnant—their periods are late and they experience the effects of heightened hormones. A sonogram alone is not enough to diagnose this issue, because during the first trimester of pregnancy, the ruptured follicle stays on the surface of the ovary (we call this the corpus luteum, see page 14) to produce sustaining hormones (primarily progesterone). So first, the doctor will do a pregnancy test to discount that possibility and then a sonogram to examine the cyst.

In the sixties and up to the mid seventies, early pregnancy tests were very costly and not very accurate (there was the rat to pay for, see page 147). Progesterone was a crude pregnancy test. If a patient's period was late, and she was given progesterone for ten days, she would only get her period if she weren't pregnant. If she didn't, she was.

How we treat this problem depends on the patient's needs. If this is an isolated event, she can ride it out and see if she gets her period the following month. Ninety percent of the time she'll get her period and return to menstrually normal. Another choice would be to briefly take progesterone, mimicking ovulation, and the cessation of this hormone will cause the uterine lining to shed. This restarts the menstrual cycle.

Hemhorragic Functional Cysts

If, at the site of the follicle rupture, there is a small vein or artery that also ruptures, it will cause the patient to bleed internally. Symptoms of this include severe abdominal pain and distension. As you're bleeding, you might feel light-headed and fainting is common. These symptoms also mimic a ruptured ectopic pregnancy (see page 206), and the way to distinguish between the two is the pregnancy test.

This is extraordinarily rare, and it is one of the few times that functional cysts call for surgery. It's a relatively simple procedure, depending on how much blood is in the patient's abdomen. If it's not too much, this can be done quickly and laproscopically (i.e. with a really small, not terribly invasive instrument). Otherwise, a simple bikini-line incision is made for the surgeon to stitch the vessel that's bleeding.

Large Functional Cysts

Ninety-five percent of cysts under five centimeters in diameter are functional, which gives the gynecologist a certain confidence about

significant problems of the ovaries and fallopian tubes

195

waiting and watching relatively small cysts. However, when cysts are larger than five centimeters, the percentage of those that are still functional drops 10 or 20 percent. This is not as comforting a statistic, and usually doctors handle these more aggressively, suggesting surgery much sooner. If doctors had a way to prove that these large growths were functional, without operating, they would surely do so. Even so, large functional cysts are almost always an incidental finding of a sonogram or pelvic exam, as they are asymptomatic.

Polycystic Ovaries

Polycystic ovaries defy classification—they are a functional aberration of the ovary, which is not a cause for significant medical concern. Like the name suggests, polycystic ovaries are ovaries that make a lot of follicles that never rupture and ovulation never happens; meanwhile, each follicle stays on the surface of the ovary and makes hormones.

This dysfunctional environment creates an excess of both male and female hormones, which classically caused obesity, acne, and outrageous hair growth. Additionally, the patient would generally menstruate infrequently (called oligomenorhea) if at all, and she could develop insulin resistance that contributes to her obesity.

Today, doctors can diagnose polycystic ovaries by monitoring subtle changes in hormone ratios that are determined through a blood test. It also helps to have a sonogram where one can see the multiple unruptured follicles on the ovaries.

Polycystic ovaries are like a skipping record—your ovaries keep doing what they think they're supposed to be doing, when in fact they're only doing the same thing over and over again. Treating this condition is like trying to get the needle to jump to the next track, allowing the music to continue as usual. Therefore and unsurprisingly, the standard of care for polycystic ovaries is to suppress the ovary with the birth control pill, ceasing all follicle development. When and if the patient comes off the pill, the hope is that she simply will not develop this problem again and will return to a normal, fertile menstrual cycle. The vast majority do.

In the past, I have told students with menstrual irregularities that they cannot be overly concerned until they are out of college. All the social and academic pressures of a university environment, coupled with their proximity to adolescence, can be very stressful on a woman's reproductive cycle. It's not uncommon for women in their early twenties to skip periods occasionally, or to suffer corollary hormone imbalances, including acne and weight gain. Six periods a year is the fewest that you can safely do nothing about.

Of course, this tactic is not attractive for a woman who is trying to get pregnant. These women are generally prescribed an antiestrogen called Clomid, which reduces the estrogen level to the point where the pituitary will jump in and restart a normal menstrual cycle. Frequently, a diabetic medication is also prescribed to treat the patient's insulin resistance.

Despite it's scary-sounding name, polycystic ovaries can be directly related to lifestyle. In fact, polycystic ovaries can be diagnosed at such a relatively early or mild stage, that often the problem can be corrected through simple behavioral adjustments. For example, if an overathletic woman ceases to menstruate for three months, a sonogram might reveal what look like polycystic ovaries. She may have no physical symptoms. While Chlomid or the birth control pill might help with her lack of ovulation and her polycystic condition, reducing her athletic activities might yield equally good results.

Malignant vs. Benign
Sometimes a first sonogram conclusively reveals a nonfunctional cyst. This happens when the growth is solid or if there's a tooth in it (see page 199). If you have two sonograms and the cyst is in the same location and growing, this also demonstrates conclusively that it is not functional.

significant problems of the ovaries and fallopian tubes

197

At least half-a-dozen patients have come in to my office practically wearing tents, they've grown so large. I say, "Your abdominal cavity is filled with a mass of some kind," and they respond with things like, "I thought I was gaining weight." or "I thought I just needed to work out." These are intelligent women who, for reasons of denial or thoughtlessness, allowed an unidentified growth to grow unchecked to the point where it fills their abdominal cavity. There's a famous gynecological textbook picture from a hundred years ago of a woman who needed a wheelbarrow to carry her ovarian growth around with her. Any ovarian abnormality has the potential to grow indefinitely—so if you gain a whole lot of weight exclusively in your gut, it may not be the double-stuff Oreos. Get it checked out.

These are tumors unrelated to ovulation-like tumors that can grow anywhere else in the body. At this point, your doctor should focus her energy on answering the question, "Is it benign or malignant?" The only way to answer that question is through a biopsy, which is where a physician removes some or all of the growth and a pathologist looks at it under a microscope. This can be done through abdominal surgery or a laproscopic biopsy. This also depends on the skill and experience of your doctor, who may have her preferred method.

These kinds of growths, both benign and malignant, are usually discovered by happenstance. During a routine exam, a gynecologist might feel a mass on the ovary. A physician performing abdominal surgery on a woman can also check on those pesky ovaries and make sure they're not up to any mischief, although this is not standard. And sometimes a sonogram for another problem will reveal an ovarian growth.

There are many kinds of benign growths of the ovary, but they all pose a danger to the ovary itself because they have a tendency to grow. They do not invade neighboring organs (like cancer) but they press in a persistent and damaging fashion. Much as water dripping on a stone can eventually drill through rock, benign ovarian growths can compress neighboring healthy ovarian tissue, ultimately killing it. So in general, these growths need to come out, even though they are not life threatening. This approach should obviously be tailored to the patient; a woman over fifty who's finished with childbearing might elect to simply have the whole ovary removed and spare herself any future visits to the operating room for a recurrent tumor. Meanwhile, surgeons work to protect the ovaries of women who still desire children.

BENIGN OVARIAN TUMORS

Dermoid Cysts

Amongst young women, the most common cystic tumor is a benign cystic teratoma, or, in slang, a *dermoid* cyst. This is a cyst that originates from an egg that inexplicably divides without the influence of a sperm. They are one of our bodies harmless, mysterious idiosyncrasies, that only cause a problem if left unchecked. These days, physicians often catch these when they are too small to worry about, usually by happening upon them (e.g. a pelvic sonogram for something else reveals a dermoid).

Gross or Cool; You Decide

....

Three stem cells (ectoderm, mesoderm, and endoderm) develop into the entire human body. The ectoderm becomes the skeleton, the mesoderm grows into guts and muscles, and the endoderm morphs into skin and hair. Sperm comprises half of the process of human reproduction, but picture a lone, renegade egg dividing on its own. This is a dermoid. True to its triptych roots, the dermoid is characterized by the presence of fat (mesoderm), hair (endoderm), and, most fascinatingly, a tooth (ectoderm). Before sonograms, physicians would diagnose this with a simple X-ray, which would often reveal a fully formed tooth.

....

These days, sonography is so excellent, we can see one centimeter cysts—sometimes in the middle of the ovary. These growths are so small, it would be more damaging to extract them than to leave them where they are. For these women, a physician could recommend biannual sonograms to make sure the dermoid doesn't grow.

Miscellaneous Benign Ovarian Tumors

Tumors occur when a normal cell mutates into something that can either be benign or malignant but is always intent on dividing and growing. Most tumors are defined by the first cell to mutate and begin growing out of control. Benign tumor cells look much like the cells they came from, while cancerous cells can be extraordinarily different (in medicine, we call this *anaplastic*). In the ovary, there are essentially three kinds of cells that can become tumors: cells associated with the follicle (like a dermoid), cells on the surface of the ovary, and cells associated with the connective tissue of the ovary, or the stroma. Each of these three types spawn even further myriad potential tumors.

Among these kinds of tumors, there is a spectrum of benign to malignant. Some are definitely benign, others definitely malignant,

Proper Names

While we are lumping many benign ovarian tumors into one group, your physician will use a specific diagnosis, especially if (when!) you ask. These names include *fibroma*, *cystadenoma*, *mucinous cystadenoma*, *paraovarian* cyst, and many more. All of these types of tumors (except endometriomas, which are often indicative of endometriosis; see page 221) have the same symptoms, health implications, and treatment options. They all have an incidence of recurrence and bilaterality (they can recur later on the same or other ovary), meaning that it's very important to know exactly what kind of cyst you may have. If you switch physicians, and your new physician discovers a pelvic mass, it would be very helpful for her to know what she's likely to be dealing with.

Endometrioma is a cyst on the ovary resulting from endometriosis (a uterine problem, see page 221). These cysts fill with blood, which lingers and oxidizes, developing the consistency of chocolate syrup. That's why endometriomas of the ovary are colloquially called chocolate cysts.

and a few are "borderline," or of low malignant potential. Therefore, it's standard practice to remove all ovarian growths, except for well-documented, small, stable dermoids and endometriomas. The many benign tumors of the ovary are all uncommon, but nonetheless have to be looked at under a microscope.

Some ovarian tumors produce hormones, all of which must be removed because they have the potential to be malignant, and even if they're not, they're still damaging. This is sometimes hard to catch in an adult female, but in a prepubertal girl, the estrogen-producing cystic tumor announces itself by causing girls as young as five to grow breasts and menstruate. Even more disconcerting, the tumor can produce the male hormone testosterone. This causes the unsuspecting owner to grow a moustache, develop a lower voice, and a larger clitoris (called *clitoromegaly*). A particular kind of dermoid can make thyroid hormone, producing the symptoms of an overactive thyroid, even though the patient's problem is on her ovary.

OVARIAN CANCER

Since an ovary floats freely in the abdomen, should cancer develop, there's no surface layer to contain the disease. The organ has the potential to shed malignant cells very quickly, which can then roam all over the abdominal cavity. Despite this dramatic sounding process, ovarian cancer gives few signs that it is there. This disease is therefore diagnosed at a later stage with fewer treatment options than most other cancers.

significant problems of the ovaries and fallopian tubes

201

From a Doctor's Perspective

Ovarian cancer is the worst disease I deal with. Some women are forced to walk a very fine line between fertility and death. Women love to have children, and with good reason. It's good, fun, rewarding—it's our joy. But for some unfortunates, there's a choice to be made between that potential baby and the very real risk that they are taking with their lives. For example, I luckily discovered early ovarian cancer in a patient, and she had both her ovaries removed. She was young and had recently married, so her oncologist and I agreed that she could keep her uterus if she chose to, after fully understanding the risks. This is *not* the standard of care—gynecologic oncologists have found that removing the uterus, tubes, and ovaries is the best way to guarantee survival. However, this patient subsequently carried two children thanks to an egg donor.

Symptoms for ovarian cancer are virtually nonexistent, and even as the disease progresses, it can be nearly impossible to identify. A famous patient of mine had three homes, East Coast, West Coast, and Europe. I was her New York doctor—not an optimal medical situation. Everyone should have one primary doctor to quarterback all your medical care. Her English doctor diagnosed her general symptoms (abdominal discomfort, fatigue, malaise, "I don't feel well") as a virus.

In New York, she told me that she was still not feeling great, which was strange. Things in her life were going so well, she didn't know why she was so tired. I recommended another ultrasound. The radiologist said her pelvis looked hazy and abnormal, but he couldn't make out a tumor. I told her she needed another laparoscopy, since there was something wrong. She said, "Okay, I'll get it done in California."

I never saw her again. She passed away from widespread ovarian cancer two years later. She had a particularly nasty kind of cancer where the ovaries shed malignant cells, causing multiple little tumors throughout the abdomen while the ovary itself stays normal in size. It turned out that she had what is called hereditary ovarian cancer—most of the women in her family had died of the disease.

There is a subset of ovarian cancer that is a dominant, genetically inherited trait, called hereditary ovarian cancer. This accounts for 10 percent of all incidences of the disease. It is possible to test for the presence of a gene that is linked to ovarian and breast cancer, called the Brca-1 or Brca-2 gene, though both are more commonly associated with breast cancer. If you have one of these genes, it is appropriate for you to finish having children and get rid of those ovaries as soon as possible. In the absence of the Brca-1 or Brca-2 gene, a family medical history of ovarian cancer can still dictate major health decisions. Since this particular disease is so difficult to detect at an early stage and highly fatal, a patient who has one or two immediate family members (a mother, sister, or daughter) with ovarian cancer will often be advised to remove her ovaries as soon as she has finished childbearing and to keep an eye on them sonographically in the meantime. And an unfortunate woman who has seen three immediate family members battle ovarian cancer must consider removing her ovaries immediately.

For the average woman, however, the standard of care for the detection of ovarian disease is the annual pelvic exam. Many clinicians and scientists have devoted time and energy to developing the ability to diagnose ovarian cancer earlier. Routine vaginal ultrasounds or blood tests have shown no change in the mortality rate thus far. With breast cancer, if you get a normal mammogram today and in a year there is an abnormality, the odds are overwhelming that you're still at a very early stage of the disease. If you have a normal vaginal ultrasound today, in a year you could have advanced ovarian cancer.

The only scientific indicator we currently have for ovarian cancer is a blood test that I use and recommend with caution because it is sketchy and inconclusive. The CA125 blood test reads as elevated 50 percent of the time for actual ovarian cancer. However, it can also read

significant problems of the ovaries and fallopian tubes

203

A new blood test for ovarian cancer is due to be released any day now, if it hasn't already been. Called Ova Check, the advance reports on this blood test show it to be highly accurate at early detection of ovarian cancer. The gynecological community is very hopeful about this new diagnostic tool, but it is not proven yet. Keep your ears open for news on this exciting development.

as elevated for benign problems, like fibroids and endometriosis. This means that if you are premenopausal, went to your gynecologist with vague symptoms, asked her for this test, and it came back elevated, it wouldn't help to diagnose you. The CA125 is a somewhat more useful tool for postmenopausal women because at that point endometriosis and fibroids are inactive, so an elevation is much more likely to represent an ovarian malignancy.

For premenopausal women, the chances of ovarian cancer are quite small, as cancer in general is an older person's problem. The median age of ovarian cancer detection in the United States is fifty-nine, though the median age for women with hereditary ovarian cancer is forty-nine. Your best defense is to stay faithful to your annual gynecological exam, and if your doctor should recommend tests or follow-up visits, don't be lazy.

MISCELLANEOUS OVARIAN PROBLEMS

Abscesses are another structural abnormality of the ovary that form as healthy tissue fights bacteria. These are essentially sacs of white blood cells that congregate around an intruding infection: in other words, big pus globs. This is the end result of untreated pelvic inflammatory disease (PID, see page 107).

Abscesses are frequently secondary to gonorrhea and chlamydia. When a patient catches a sexually transmitted disease such as gonohrrea, the infection lives very happily for a time on the cervix. When the patient menstruates, the blood feeds the bacteria, which then divide like crazy. Following the trail of food like bread crumbs, the bacteria heads up into the uterus. Then the period ends and the bugs go crazy looking for food, straight out the fallopian tubes. Thus the major symptom of this particular condition is severe pelvic pain, right after a period, usually accompanied by a high fever. If you ever have a significant temperature and severe pain between your belly button and your pubic bone, contact your gynecologist immediately.

Ovarian mechanical problems can be another cause of extreme abdominal pain. The ovary is suspended on a ligament that contains its blood supply. This ligament can twist for unknown reasons, cutting off the ovary's life support system. When there's no blood to a part of your body, there is dying. No blood to the brain = brain damage. No blood to the ovary = ovary damage. The pain can be excruciating as the ovary screams in agony because it's being deprived of its blood flow.

A healthy, twisted ovary is very, very rare. But once there's a tumor or large cyst on the ovary, it may give it more torque and

Ovarian Sparing

Should you need radiation treatments in your abdomen, your ovaries will be jeopardized. There are cancer centers that will remove your ovaries and put them somewhere else in your body away from the radiation. The ovaries can live anywhere with a blood supply, and from their new neighborhood they can continue to supply you with all the hormones you need. Currently, scientists are working on honing their ability to extract eggs from these ovaries and freezing them so that these patients can still be biological mothers. New approaches also include removing and freezing all or part of an ovary, reimplanting it in the patient after she is cured, and then trying to extract eggs from it. So if you are still of reproductive age and may undergo medical care that can injure your ovaries, inquire about ovarian sparing techniques.

encourage this problem. This is another reason to remove any ovarian growth.

If you do not seek treatment, eventually gangrene (i.e. rotting) may set in. Gangrene in your abdomen will make you very, very sick. Don't writhe in pain at home—go to the emergency room or call your doctor should you experience this kind of mind-blowing pain.

FALLOPIAN TUBES

ECTOPIC PREGNANCY

The most dangerous complication related to the fallopian tubes is the ectopic (i.e. out-of-place) pregnancy, or any pregnancy that progresses outside of the uterus. This happens in about one in sixty pregnancies. The most common (99 percent) is the tubal pregnancy, so these terms are used interchangeably. Very rarely, a fertilized egg can land in the abdominal cavity somewhere, on a loop of intestine or a big artery. It's a very dangerous medical situation when a fertilized egg implants anywhere other than the endometrium, because the uterus is

Pelvic Infections of the Caribbean

· ·

When I did a year of my residency in Jamaica, the ectopic pregnancy rate was approximately 5 percent. This is very high, and it was mostly due to ineffective treatment of bacterial STDs. Women would come in with PID, very sick, their abdominal cavities full of pus and with massive infections. We treated them with aggressive antibiotics for twenty-four hours, and discharged them with a prescription for oral antibiotics. But many could not afford the pills, and therefore would or could not take them. So ultimately, they had just enough medicine to keep the tubes from closing entirely. The passage was still wide enough for sperm to reach an egg and fertilize it, but not enough for the fertilized egg (a larger mass than the sperm) to get back down to the uterus. The lesson here is always, always, always finish a course of antibiotics.

· ·

Emergency Room Tip

....

Just consider that if you are of reproductive age, are sexually active,
and have severe abdominal pain, a complication of pregnancy should
be considered as part of your medical picture.

....

the only suitable place for a pregnancy to grow (and grow and grow).
Should the pregnancy land in the tubes, the embryo will soon out-
grow the small tube, causing it to burst, which leads to massive internal bleeding.

Ectopic pregnancies can happen to anyone, but usually, they are
a direct result of scarring from previous infections. The major
offenders here are sexually transmitted diseases like chlamydia and
gonorrhea, which do quick damage to the tubes. If caught soon
enough, these diseases are easy to cure without causing permanent
scarring, but when they are left untreated, they can lead to tubal
obstructions or blockage.

Most dangerous is partial scarring, which causes ectopic pregnancies. This happens when the tube is open enough for the sperm to swim
out to the egg at the outer third of the tube, but when the fertilized egg
swims back to implant, it hits a scar or an obstruction of some kind.
This teeny four-cell zygote doesn't have the ability to back up and go
around the obstruction. It keeps batting its body against that scar until
it's time to implant, at which point, it will do so wherever it is. Less life
threatening, but still significantly life altering is when the tubes are
completely blocked due to scarring. This causes infertility, which
mechanically comparable to tubal ligation (see page 95).

Ectopic pregnancies are the greatest cause of mortality associated
with pregnancy in this country because they are easily overlooked. If
an ectopic lodges in the narrowest stretch of your tube, it can rupture
before you're even late for your period. Typically, the patient is a day or
two late, has sudden severe abdominal pain, and rushes to the

significant problems of the ovaries and fallopian tubes

207

emergency room. It has to occur to the physician to do a pregnancy test immediately, even though she could arguably assume any number of other problems.

* * * * *

MOTHER: "I hate ovaries."

DAUGHTER: "Stop whining."

MOTHER: "You don't know. There are dozens of tumors of the ovaries. One in a million this, one in a trillion that."

DAUGHTER: "But you have to kind of like ovaries too."

MOTHER: "Why?"

DAUGHTER: "Because they keep you in business."

chapter thirteen

SIGNIFICANT PROBLEMS OF THE UTERUS

\his-'ter-ē-ə\, n. A nervous affection, occurring almost exclusively in women, in which the emotional and reflex excitability is exaggerated, and the willpower correspondingly diminished, so that the patient loses control over the emotions, becomes the victim of imaginary sensations, and often falls into paroxism or fits. From Greek word hystera, meaning womb.

—*Webster's Revised Unabridged Dictionary*

I found this definition in March 2004, at www.dictionary.com. It's ironic that the information superhighway could yield such a seemingly antiquated point of view, but there it is.

The uterus is a hollow, muscular organ of multiple parts and is primarily used during pregnancy. Today, women don't get pregnant nearly as much as we used to, so the medical community pays much more attention to the nonpregnant uterus than ever before.

Within the uterus, there are the cervix, the endometrium, and the myometrium (see page 3). The cervix is the gateway to the uterus, keeping out foreign invaders that run rampant in the vagina. In a healthy situation, the uterine cavity is sterile, meaning there are no viruses or bacteria. The endometrium lines the uterus and is shed every month in the absence of pregnancy. The myometrium is the muscular layer at the top of the uterus that stretches in pregnancy, and contracts to expel either menstrual fluid or products of reproduction, including babies.

THINGS THAT CAN HAPPEN TO THE MYOMETRIUM
FIBROIDS

Within the myometrium, whorls of fibrous tissue can form, called leiomyomata, or fibroids. Like freckles, women rarely have just one. These benign tumors consist of smooth muscle and extracellular material, such as collagen. Fibroids are estrogen dependent, which means that they shrink at menopause. While they are usually considered relatively innocuous, they can compromise the patient's quality of life and cause problems in labor. Fibroids are extraordinarily common, and are the number one nonmalignant cause of hysterectomies in the United States.

Fibroids occur in upwards of 80 percent of women usually past the age of thirty-five. The vast majority go unnoticed and never cause the patient any harm. Thirty percent of women have fibroids that lead to noticeable symptoms.

Fibroids can be big or small, grow quickly or slowly, and are found all over the uterus. Forget fruit comparisons ("It's as big as a grapefruit!") today fibroids are sized by volume, measured sonographically and equated to the size of pregnancy. A "ten-week-sized-fibroid uterus" means that the fibroid plus the uterus is the equivalent of a ten-week pregnancy. However, like real estate, with fibroids location is everything.

SUBSEROSAL FIBROIDS

Fibroids can be on the outside of your uterus (the serosa) and continue to grow outward. These are called subserosal fibroids. They can be very large, grow very quickly, and are asymptomatic, which means physicians usually happen upon them while looking for something else. While a sonogram that reveals a big, solid tumor in the abdomen is distressing, the subserosal fibroid is not of much medical concern (if it is certainly a fibroid). However, physicians generally recommend removing susberosal fibroids for women who intend on getting pregnant, as they can twist and degenerate. This is not dangerous to the pregnancy, as much as it is potentially painful to the mother (see page 215).

INTRAMURAL FIBROIDS

The intramural fibroid grows within the wall of the uterus, causing the uterine muscles to stretch around the fibroid, like rocks in a stream. This may worsen menstrual cramps, but the intramural fibroid does not present a significant health problem. The only issue is the functionality of the uterus in labor—will it contract effectively, both during labor and afterwards to stave blood loss? The unlikely danger is dysfunctional labor and postpartum hemorrhaging. These risks are completely unpredictable.

SUBMUCOUS FIBROID

The submucous fibroid accounts for approximately 5 percent of all fibroids and is of medical significance, though it is treatable. This fibroid bulges into the cavity of the uterus, stretching the endometrium, and impeding the local blood vessels from contracting during menstruation. This kind of fibroid can cause severe, prolonged, heavy periods, resulting in persistent anemia. While all fibroids can compete with the baby for room and food, the submucous fibroid is the most immediate threat.

PEDUNCULATED FIBROIDS

Rarely, a fibroid can grow on a pedicle (i.e. attached to the uterus by a stem) and twist on its stalk (as with the ovaries, see page 205). These are not particularly threatening to pregnancy or the woman's health, except in rare cases where the fibroid turns (for no good reason). The twisting of the stem compresses the artery, cutting off that all-important, life-support system. The fibroid then rots due to lack of oxygen. This can cause considerable pain, and if gangrene sets in, the patient's health is in danger. Luckily, pendunculated fibroids are the easiest to remove, carrying a very low risk of hysterectomy or extensive blood loss.

significant problems of the uterus

I had a patient whose sonogram, when she was five months pregnant, revealed a large solid mass to the right of the uterus. The radiologist was very concerned, as he could not see any attachment between the uterus and the growth, even though it looked like a fibroid. This was very ominous, as it was a possible ovarian tumor. A rule of obstetrics is never to operate on fibroids during pregnancy (see page 215) because the bleeding is virtually unstoppable. But because we couldn't figure out what it was, we had to perform surgery. I made a little incision over the tumor and reached in to feel whether or not there was an attachment. There was, we stitched her up, she had a healthy baby and still has that same fibroid today.

PARASITIC FIBROIDS

These fibroids begin as pedunculated fibroids, which very rarely stretch out into the abdomen and attach to another place (e.g. a loop of bowel, the aorta, or the sidewall of the abdominal cavity). The fibroid can live off the blood supply of whatever it has attached to, and the initial stem to the uterus disappears. This is called a parasitic fibroid and is often removed because the physician usually has no idea what it is. It's no longer attached to the uterus and, on a sonogram, appears to be an unidentified solid tumor.

Treatment

What you do about fibroids depends on the symptoms, the location, your location and your doctor. If you can ride it out until menopause, then the lack of estrogen will usually shrink them. The only cure for fibroids premenopausally is surgery. The indications for surgery are bleeding to anemia that you cannot correct, rapid growth of the fibroid, and ureteral compression (preventing the urine from flowing freely between the kidney and bladder).

There are also relative indications for surgery-meaning it's not absolutely, universally necessary, but a patient's particular situation may call for it. For instance, a woman who is forced to live in the bathroom because a fibroid is pressing on her bladder may understandably consider surgery. Or a fibroid can press on the rectum, giving her either constant urgency or persistent constipation. Or a fibroid can make intercourse uncomfortable. Or a woman with a very bulbous fibroid can look five or six months pregnant. These are all significant inconveniences that make surgery an attractive option.

Once a woman and her physician decide on surgery, there are still multiple choices. A myomectomy is when the surgeon shells out (like a pea) the fibroid through an incision in the uterus, and then reapproximates (i.e. reconstructs) the uterine wall.

At first blush, this sounds like an attractive option. However, this is a difficult procedure because fibroids are usually multiple and bloody. Worst of all, one myomectomy generally does not do the trick; those pesky fibroids have a nasty habit of coming back. In 90 percent of patients with four or more fibroids, the little devils recurred after surgery. Myomectomies are three times more likely to require a blood transfusion and in general, carry a higher infection rate than hysterectomies. Three percent of myomectomies result in hysterectomies anyway, because when the surgeon removes all the fibroids sometimes there isn't much uterus left. Also, should the patient hemorrhage during a myomectomy, a hysterectomy can become necessary to save her life. Regardless, if you need to treat your fibroids surgically, myomectomies are the only choice for women who want more children. For women who are done having children, a hysterectomy is a simpler, more effective solution.

A newer approach to treating fibroids is vascular embolization. This was originally attempted when the patient was too sick and anemic to undergo surgery, so a radiologist suggested passing a catheter through the groin to destroy the artery feeding the fibroid. This applies the concept of the twisted fibroid (the fibroid dies due to lack of blood) and can be similarly painful. As the fibroid rots, the patient can experience severe pain, to the point where she may find herself in the emergency room a few times for medication. Also, the blood vessel that supplies the fibroid may additionally supply muscles, which will also die during this process. This is currently not an option for women who want more children; because the procedure is so new, it is impossible to gauge the risk of pregnancy after this procedure. Doctors theorize that it could compromise the muscles required for effective contractions or contribute to a ruptured uterus during pregnancy.

Medication is also an option for treating fibroids, though not a long-term solution. GnRH (gonadotropin releasing hormone) agonist (brand name Lupron) fights the hormone that stimulates the pituitary to stimulate the ovary to make hormones. This is administered as a monthly shot and will suppress ovarian function, putting the patient into a psuedo menopausal state, thereby shrinking the fibroids. Unfortunately, Lupron is unpredictable. It's impossible to tell how much a particular patient's fibroids will shrink, and how long does any young woman want to stay menopausal, anyway? For the period on this medication, the patient loses bone mass, has hot flashes, suffers vaginal atrophy, and all of the other myriad symptoms of menopause, and no woman should go through that twice, or, arguably, even once.

Typically, Lupron is used as a temporary treatment. For example, before surgery, women often go on Lupron to shrink a large fibroid and reduce its blood supply. Additionally, they cease menstruating, which reduces their anemia and builds up their red blood cells for surgery. The downside to preoperative Lupron is that smaller fibroids can disappear entirely, so your physician might have trouble finding them in surgery even though they are still there, waiting for their opportunity to blossom again. Preoperative Lupron is therefore ideal for women who are having hysterectomies, because it shrinks the uterus and reduces blood loss.

Pregnancy and Fibroids

Pregnancy and fibroids are a risky combination for a variety of reasons. It's not that catastrophic things tend to happen when one is pregnant and has fibroids, but rather that they tend to cause a more difficult

vaginas

I sit down with my patient and we examine her particular situation together. If her fibroids are quite large and in an inopportune place, I generally recommend a myomectomy before pregnancy. If we decide that the fibroids are not so significant, we do nothing. The patient gets pregnant, and we hopefully breeze through without any problems, which happens most of the time.

pregnancy overall. The blood supply that would usually just feed the baby also has to keep pace with a rapidly growing fibroid—it's like having twins. You are more likely to have preterm labor or discomfort, and during delivery, you are more likely to have higher blood loss. There is also the possibility that a fibroid can block the baby's way out of the uterus, and in those cases, a cesarean section is mandated.

Among the more drastic things that can go wrong with fibroids in pregnancy is that they begin to degenerate due to lack of food—sometimes the baby wins out for the blood supply. It may sound like good news, but actually, this causes the center of the fibroid to rot. This is extremely painful, and these women are generally admitted into the hospital and put on pain medication that is not harmful to the baby.

Unfortunately, prepregnancy fibroid surgery is not a very attractive option. Myomectomies cause some uterine scarring, which are like fault lines in the wall of the organ—they could split at a very inopportune time. If the scar permeates the thickness of the uterine wall, the patient must have a cesarean section. Also, myomectomies can, out of emergent necessity, become hysterectomies in the operating room. Some women choose to take Lupron temporarily, but the hormones of pregnancy stimulate fibroids to grow faster than ever.

significant problems of the uterus

215

In certain parts of the United States, up through the 1970s and possibly into the eighties, women from a certain socioeconomic background who went to the hospital with abdominal pain and were deemed less bright or disabled in any way would receive surgery and end up infertile. Eugenicist physicians would take the surgical opportunity to disrupt the reproductive system of these unfortunate women. This was so common it has its own alliterative moniker (brace yourself!)—the Alabama appendectomy.

Hysterectomies—A Mixed Bag

Hysterectomies are a deceivingly simple concept—this is surgery to remove the uterus. However, there are several different approaches to the procedure, and twice as many opinions and feelings about it.

Medical dogma, hospital policies, attitudes about the uterus, how your doctor was trained, and countless other factors can contribute to what you may hear from your physician with regard to removing your uterus. In certain medical communities, if you already have a few children, you may be asked: "What do you need your uterus for?" There are also regions where doctors tend to recommend hysterectomies much more freely—for fibroids, cramps, or heavy periods, for example. Often in these same geographic areas, women have children at a younger age, meaning that a hysterectomy can be convenient birth control. In some ways, this attitude has its upside. Without a uterus, a woman never has to worry about cervical cancer, endometrial cancer, fibroids, cramps, bleeding, anemia, etc. Of course, the patient must be absolutely certain that she never wants to have any or another child.

On the flip side, some women (and a good chunk of my patients) will hold onto their uteri in the face of severe anemia, massive fibroids, and borderline illnesses. This is another case of politics and fashion entering medicine, which rarely does anyone any good health-wise.

There's an appropriate balance here. The uterus is an organ that can be diseased and may need removal. On the other hand, this is a significant surgery with long-term implications. It should not be undertaken lightly.

Once you decide on the hysterectomy, there are further choices to make. As with so many other forks in the gynecological road, which way a woman goes depends on what she prefers, where she is in the world, the disease her doctor is treating, and whether a surgeon or gynecologist will perform the procedure.

Abdominal Hysterectomies

In this approach, the surgeon makes a four- to six-inch abdominal incision and removes the uterus and traditionally, the cervix. If the surgery is for a benign problem, the incision can be horizontal and in the pubic hair (known as a bikini-line incision) , which becomes virtually invisible within a year. Unfortunately, if the surgery is for most malignant problems, the doctor will want to make a vertical incision from the pubic bone to the belly button, with the understanding that, should the need arise, the incision might grow longer.

Typically, patients take six weeks to fully recover from an abdominal hysterectomy. The major postoperative symptom is fatigue, as the body focuses all its energy on the healing process. There's no significant pain, but in the first two weeks after surgery, these women are simply too tired to get around much. Their abdomens have been profoundly disturbed, so bowel movements can be disrupted. After four weeks, patients start considering vacations and dinners out. This is not to say that women have never returned to work after a week, but they are heroic, stoic females. Count on at least a month off with an option to renew.

Currently, the uterus can be removed without the cervix, though this depends on the patient's particular situation. Removing the whole uterus (including the cervix) became fashionable in the 1960s to the point that it was widely considered the only appropriate hysterectomy. Prior to the development of routine Pap smears, if a woman developed

There are women who claim tremendous sexual pleasure when the cervix is directly hit with the thrusting penis (or whatever else). Even though it's been mentioned on *Sex and the City*, it still isn't a well-studied response. However, many women who have had their uteri and/or cervixes removed claim that their sexual pleasure is diminished. For these reasons, when possible, surgeons will offer a subtotal hysterectomy, preserving the cervix, and removing the top half of the uterus. Also, the cervix provides much of the support for the vaginal chamber. Without it, patients run the risk of future vaginal prolapse (inversion).

cervical cancer and did not have a uterus, it seemed the cancer was more difficult to treat. With the advent of regular diagnostics, the cervix can often be preserved, with the understanding that the patient must see her gynecologist regularly for those life-saving Pap smears.

Vaginal Hysterectomies

Don't worry, the vagina doesn't get removed in a vaginal hysterectomy, it's just named for the route the surgeon takes. In this procedure, the physician grabs the cervix from the vagina and works up from there, eventually pulling the whole uterus and cervix out like a plug.

The recovery from a vaginal hysterectomy is easier, as there is no abdominal incision. Patients can often go home the same day, if not the next day. Nothing in the abdominal cavity is disturbed, so most of your bodily functions (e.g. bowel movements) are more likely to continue normally.

This procedure usually requires a certain laxity in the ligaments that support the uterus, something that happens naturally during pregnancy. Additionally, the vagina stretches in a vaginal delivery, so that the gynecologist can maneuver the uterus more freely. A uterus that has never carried a pregnancy is a firmly ensconced organ that may need to be removed abdominally, and a vagina that's never seen a baby is a tight passageway for this procedure.

The LAVH (laparoscopic assisted vaginal hysterectomy) is a new technique for a vaginal hysterectomy and makes it possible for some doctors to get around the surgery's previous limitations. A laparoscope is a small instrument that, with minimal invasion (it is inserted through a quarter-inch incision in the belly button) allows surgeons to look inside the abdominal cavity and perform many of the same operations, without a big incision. In an LAVH, the laproscope is inserted through the belly button, allowing the surgeon to cut all the attachments of the uterus to the body, and then the doctor can remove the cervix and uterus through the vagina. The advantage of this method is that it can be readily performed on women regardless of whether or not they have had children.

Vaginal vs. Abdominal

With a vaginal hysterectomy, the cervix is lost, but there is no abdominal incision and postoperative recovery is easier. With the abdominal approach, the cervix and vagina remain the same. Also, a surgeon can

What About the Ovaries?

In a hysterectomy, only the uterus is implicated. For benign disorders, the ovaries and tubes are a topic that must be discussed very specifically by both patient and doctor when they are planning a hysterectomy. Many argue that there is no reason to leave ovaries in a postmenopausal woman. In a woman over forty-five (the average menopause is around fifty), the current standard is to remove the ovaries as well, to spare this patient the risk of deadly ovarian cancer. Under forty-five, the physician should try to leave the ovaries where they are. However, this is again more often than not a personal choice; what is the patient's philosophy on HRT, her feelings about her ovaries, her risk of ovarian cancer, etc?

see the entire abdominal cavity, giving her the opportunity to visually evaluate all of the internal organs, reproductive and nonreproductive alike. The choice is generally the patient's, except in the case of a malignancy. For uterine and ovarian cancer, the standard of care is a total abdominal hysterectomy, which means the cervix, ovaries, and tubes all go. For cervical cancer, sometimes the ovaries can remain in the abdomen, churning out their all-important hormones.

SARCOMA

Sarcoma is cancer of the smooth muscle, which in this case is the myometrium. Sarcomas account for less than 10 percent of uterine malignancies. Sarcomas frequently arise in uteri that already have fibroids, but they are discreet entities—i.e. currently, doctors believe fibroids almost never become malignant. All sarcomas have the potential for aggressive biological behavior, but the range of virulence is dramatic. The only way for a physician to suspect a sarcoma is when a sonogram shows rapid enlargement of a uterine mass, particularly after menopause.

Radiation Mistakes (and We're not Talking about Chernobyl)

When I was a teenager, I had a small breakout problem. My father, Dr. Joe Livoti, sent me to a dermatologist, who said, "Oh, too bad. We only just stopped giving radiation for acne." In retrospect, this was part of a trend in medicine to radiate many benign problems or even no problems at all. Children returning from camp with ringworm were given radiation to the scalp. As a gimmick, shoe stores had small open X-ray machines, where eager children could stick their feet and watch their toes wiggle to see if their shoes fit. They found that radiation shrunk fibroids, so they exposed many women's abdomens to radiation. Approximately sixteen years later, a relatively high percentage of these women developed sarcomas. Now, radiation is used sparingly and with reservations, especially for the younger patient.

When you are dealing with a medical situation that is a little hazy or subjective, like a borderline uterine tumor, it is a very good idea to request a second opinion from an alternate pathologist. It's easy to forget that pathologists, just like with every other medical specialty, come in varying degrees of skill and experience. If the diagnosis is borderline, ask your doctor about sending your slides to a super specialist or cancer center for a second opinion.

The only known contributing factor for developing sarcoma is previous pelvic radiation. The average interval between radiation and sarcoma development is sixteen years.

How a doctor treats a sarcoma is predicated by an accurate diagnosis by a pathologist, so all sarcomas must be entirely removed so that they can be looked at microscopically. If it is a virulent cancer, the doctor must remove the uterus, tubes, and ovaries. In less malignant-looking growths, sometimes called *borderline tumors*, the sarcoma might behave just like a fibroid, meaning that the uterus may be left behind if the patient still wants to have biological children.

THINGS THAT CAN HAPPEN TO THE ENDOMETRIUM

ENDOMETRIOSIS

Like an ectopic pregnancy, the lining of the uterus (the endometrium) can misplace itself. Endometriosis (i.e. ectopic endometrium) is the condition where endometrial cells are found implanted and alive on a blood source outside of the uterine cavity. For example, when these cells land on the ovary, they cause the "chocolate cyst" (see page 201). While no one knows for certain what causes this mysterious ailment, most physicians agree that it is retrograde menstruation, meaning that

significant problems of the uterus

221

Don't get us wrong, the vast majority of the time, endometriosis is not medically important. In rare cases, though, it can behave very strangely. Those little endometrial cells can travel through the blood to far-off places. There are women who get nosebleeds every month with their period because of endometrial cells in their noses. Surgeons can leave a trail of endometrial cells in the belly button after a laproscopy, which can bleed every month. Endometriosis can even invade the bladder or bowel, where it causes significant health problems.

some of the menstrual blood goes back up the tubes and out into the abdominal cavity. Every woman to some extent has retrograde menstruation; why it causes symptomatic endometriosis in some and no problem in others is yet another mystery.

Not only do these implants cause inflammation, but they bleed each month just like the lining of your uterus. Every menstrual cycle that goes by can send new endometrium to join the old. It's painful. Serious endometriosis can cause secondary scarring around the tubes and destruction of the normal architecture of your abdominal organs. Needless to say, endometriosis contributes to infertility, though so many women unknowingly have this problem and get pregnant anyway, it's impossible to calculate how much so.

The hallmark of endometriosis is premenstrual pain—meaning abdominal pain before you get your period. Doctors theorize that the patient's menstrual blood backs up into the tubes, and the endometrial implants swell and bleed. Then, as the blood expels into the vagina, the pain subsides a little. Not everyone who has pain prior to the onset of her period has this condition, but it can be a relevant data point.

A second calling card of significant endometriosis is the retroverted (i.e. tipped) or fixed uterus. As the years go by, the worsening scarring can pull the uterus down towards the back wall of the abdomen. Sometimes, the gynecologist can even feel nodules of endometriosis on the back wall of the uterus, or on the ligaments that support it. Pain during intercourse can be a problem; it hurts when a penis hits a uterus rendered unmovable by scarring. Physicians address this problem with Lupron (page 214) or the pill, which certainly help. For a patient who is in a rush (e.g. she's forty-three and wants to get pregnant) or extremely uncomfortable, an infertility specialist can surgically break up the scarring and destroy all visible endometrial implants with a laser or cautery.

While no one knows for sure how and why it happens, endometriosis is attributed to delayed childbearing. The average age of diagnosis is twenty-six. A common estimate is that 10 percent of childless women in New York City have endometriosis by the time they're

Mom's History Corner

The uterus has been classically described as antiverted and antiflexed, meaning bent forward towards the abdominal wall. Up until the fifties, women who were having trouble getting pregnant would go to their general practitioner who would tell them, "I understand why you're not getting pregnant; your uterus is tipped." This was also considered to be a cause of dysparunia (pain on intercourse), constipation, backache, depression, hangnails, etc. As you might imagine, uterine suspension (i.e. untipping the uterus) became an extraordinarily common operation.

In the latter half of the twentieth century with the advent of sonography, we discovered that 50 percent of pregnant women have tipped uteri. Turns out, the tipped uterus is really just a variation of normal, and not in and of itself a problem. It is the patient who goes through life with an antiverted uterus that suddenly tips, who is worthy of concern as there may be a disease that caused the tipping, so to speak. So there are two very different kinds of tipped uteri—congenital and acquired—with two very different medical implications.

significant problems of the uterus

223

thirty. This condition often occurs in women who have uninterrupted cyclic menstruation (i.e. no pregnancies, systemic contraception or other menstrual cessation) for five years or more. The prevailing theory by way of explanation is incessant ovulation. We were designed to be reproductively ready at puberty, and now women are waiting twenty-five years to have children. Persistent, continuous, monthly menstruation never gives the endometrium a chance to rest and stop shedding. Nor is the uterus allowed to fulfill its mission—pregnancy, which eradicates endometriosis through hormones and uterine growth.

Treating Endometriosis

As with many other gynecological problems, the pill prevents and/or helps alleviate this condition the overwhelming majority of the time. The steady supply of hormones keeps the endometrium thinner and controlled, so that there isn't enough of it to head out into the abdominal cavity looking for trouble.

Women who already have significant endometriosis can elect to have Lupron shots once a month for up to six months. This suppresses normal ovarian function completely, putting the patient into a pseudo-menopausal state, which dries up the endometrial abdominal implants, much as they would be with a natural menopause. For women with bad endometriosis, this can be a good first step before going on the pill. Women who struggle to get pregnant because of their endometriosis also should consider a bout of Lupron.

The indications for surgery to correct endometriosis are when the patient cannot tolerate other medications, or is unwilling or unable to wait six months. Laproscopically, a surgeon can destroy (by burning, lasering, or removing) all the endometrial implants, breaking up the scar tissue, thereby allowing the woman to attempt pregnancy almost immediately. This is same-day surgery that is not terribly painful, and, in the hands of good surgeon, has as good a result as Lupron.

Finally, while this is not an option for everyone, the best treatment for endometriosis in the premenopausal woman is pregnancy. First of all, there's no retrograde menstruation for nine months. Secondly, the

@vaginas

Adenomyosis happens when endometrial cells burrow into the wall of the uterus instead of seeking out a place to live in the abdomen as they do with endometriosis. This swells the uterus and generally increases the patient's menstrual bleeding and pain, as the endometrial cells bleed within the myometrium itself. Up to 20 percent of women have this condition, especially those who have had children. A sonogram will show an enlarged uterus and findings suggestive of adenonyosis. In the rare case that it is desirable or necessary, the only treatment available is a hysterectomy.

massive amount of hormones in pregnancy will obliterate the endometriosis for anywhere from one year to a lifetime. Thirdly, as the uterus grows it destroys any uncomfortable scarring. It is extremely unfortunate that endometriosis can make it much harder to conceive.

ENDOMETRIAL CANCER

Endometrial cancer is in general a highly curable disease with clear symptoms that make early detection feasible for both pre- and postmenopausal women. Approximately 10 percent of women with postmenopausal bleeding have endometrial cancer. If a premenopausal woman has prolonged bleeding (for more than twice her normal period), significant spotting between periods, or very short cycles (less than twenty-one days), her physician might consider evaluating her for endometrial disease.

One of the major concerns for the endometrium is unopposed estrogen-or, in other words, estrogen in the absence of progesterone. Many hormonal conditions can prevent ovulation and/or progesterone production. Unopposed estrogen frequently causes endometrial cancer if sustained long enough.

There are many conditions that can lead to heightened or unopposed estrogen, which in turn can contribute to endometrial cancer.

significant problems of the uterus

225

Tamoxifin is among a new class of drugs called Selective Estrogen Receptor Modulators (SERMs), which are sometimes thought of as very weak estrogens. Other SERMs include raloxifene (brandname Evista), which is used for bone loss, and clomiphine citrate (Brandname Chlomid), which is used to treat infertility. Tamoxifin aims to block estrogenic activity on the breast, but, unfortunately, stimulates estrogenic activity in the uterus, meaning that currently, breast cancer patients must accept a very slightly increased risk of endometrial cancer. We're not talking a huge increase—it goes from 0.3 to 0.6 percent. "Endometrial Cancer Risk Doubles" is a scary headline, but a 0.3 percent increase in incidence is not that much to worry about (see page 170). Tamoxifin is far more healthful than hurtful.

Obesity is a health problem for many reasons, but because fat cells make estrogen, endometrial cancer becomes a cause of concern for the overweight woman. On the other end of the spectrum, eating disorders that prevent regular ovulation are also linked to endometrial cancer; these women never ovulate and therefore never make any progesterone to balance the estrogen. Medications like Tamoxifen, which is a major tool in the treatment of breast cancer, increase your risk of endometrial cancer as well.

ENDOMETRITIS

Endometritis is an infection of the endometrium that is usually associated with the prolonged presence of a foreign body. For instance, 2 to 5 percent of IUD users come down with endometritis. About 2 percent of abortions lead to this problem, as infection can be tracked up into the uterine cavity from the vagina. Many physicians give prophylactic antibiotics with abortions and IUD insertions to avoid infection.

Symptoms of endometritis include a discharge of pus, severe pelvic pain, and a fever. This problem does not usually affect fertility because the bacteria is generally happy to stay in the endometrium, and when it does spread, it travels along the outside of the tube. This is easy to avoid, as physicians readily treat this with antibiotics. However, as with anything else, when neglected, endometritis can become a significant health risk due to scarring and abscess formation in the uterine cavity.

POLYPS

Endometrial polyps are fairly common; 50 percent of women with spotting between periods have them. These fleshy growths extend from the endometrium into the uterine cavity—these are endometrial growths that build up over time. The only symptom of a polyp is increased, irregular vaginal bleeding. These are diagnosed with a sonogram, and 99 percent of the time they are benign (in thirty years of private practice, I've seen two malignancies). But they definitely cause menstrual irregularities, and fertility experts theorize that they can make it difficult to get pregnant. We remove them with a D&C to make sure they are benign.

THE D&C

Every specialist has a procedure for which they are famous, and for the gynecologist, it is the D&C—dilatation and curettage. The dilatation refers to the dilating of the cervix with graduated instruments that resemble sticks, stretching it one step at a time until the physician can introduce a spoon-shaped instrument called a curette into the uterus. She scrapes the lining out and sends it to a pathologist.

The procedure takes fifteen minutes, but is still generally performed in an operating room setting. The patient is put to sleep, and it therefore carries the risks of general anaesthesia (less than one in ten thousand patients will not wake up). Postprocedure, patients are crampy and can feel like they are getting their period the next day.

227

Before legalized abortion, doctors terminated pregnancies with D&Cs. The blood loss was high, and it carried an increased complication and infection rate because it took a long time and a lot of scraping. The suction curettage (see page 126) was a major improvement.

While in the past, the D&C was considered therapeutic (e.g. for irregular periods), today we consider it diagnostic.* When it comes to a menstrual irregularity or polyp, the older the patient, the more readily you suggest the D&C because a twenty-year-old is very unlikely to have endometrial cancer, but a postmenopausal woman with vaginal bleeding has a 10 to 20 percent chance of a malignancy.

NEW, IMPROVED D&CS

Like laproscopes, which gynecologists increasingly use to do vaginal hysterectomies (see page 218) and tubal ligations (see page 95), the hysteroscope is a tiny video camera that is modified to look inside the uterus. Gynecologists use the hysteroscope to ensure that they actually remove everything they intended to in a D&C. Hysteroscopes aid almost all intrauterine procedures that traditionally would have called for a large abdominal incision (e.g. removing a submucus fibroid).

The endometrial biopsy is an in-office procedure that, in theory, should eliminate the need for many D&Cs. The physician passes a catheter through the cervix and suctions out some endometrial cells, which are in turn sent to the pathologist. It saves women from the unnecessary risk of anesthesia, being admitted into a hospital, an IV, etc. The drawback is that it hurts for about thirty seconds, depending on the skill of the doctor and the patient's pain threshold. Women who

*Still, many women claim that the D&C "straightens out" their menstrual cycle.

have had their cervix stretched through childbirth generally tolerate endometrial biopsies much more readily.

The endometrial biopsy is considered to be an essential diagnostic tool for women at risk for endometrial cancer and who have dysfunctional bleeding in the absence of any apparent cause (a polyp). The endometrial biopsy is also very important in diagnosing hormone imbalances in women who are having trouble conceiving. The sonogram and endometrial biopsy combined tell the gynecologist everything she needs to know about a patient who suffers menstrual irregularities, and neither require a trip to the hospital.

* * * * *

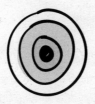

DAUGHTER: "Do you have fibroids?"

MOTHER: "No."

DAUGHTER: "How do you know?"

MOTHER: "I just don't."

DAUGHTER: "So you're one of the lucky 20 percent?"

MOTHER: "Who knows? I've never had a sonogram. I'm the only person I know who has never had one."

DAUGHTER: "Even I've had one."

MOTHER: "How do you like that?"

DAUGHTER: "Do you feel like you're missing out?"

MOTHER: "Something tells me I'm going to get a sonogram before I die, but not this month."

DAUGHTER: "What do you think you're going to get a sonogram for?"

MOTHER: "You know, if I get a new sonogram machine and want to give it a test drive."

chapter fourteen

SIGNIFICANT PROBLEMS
OF THE CERVIX

I have a friend, Katie, who's like my sister, so it's okay that she comes to me and my Mom for free medical advice and birth control pills. Recently, she called with a particularly bothersome story about a friend of hers, whose boyfriend of several years gave her HPV, which led to warts on her cervix. She met Katie for coffee and tearily relayed the whole story; how she had gone for a checkup, gotten the bad news, went for surgery, confronted her uncontrite boyfriend, who, it turns out, had known all along that he had HPV, etc. When she got to the part about the boyfriend knowingly transmitting the wart-producing virus, Katie suggested a dumping was in order. The woman responded, "But he's the last man I'll ever sleep with. I would never do this to someone else."

This is the type of silliness that keeps Dr. Phil in business. The latest research shows that HPV comes and goes within five years, and that most young, urban, singles have it. While I don't recommend going out and looking for it, should you hear the letters H-P-V from your doctor, it's not the end of the world. And staying in a relationship because you have matching STDs is ridiculous.

The cervix is the gatekeeper between the world of your uterus and the world at large. As the firm neck of the womb, the cervix and its ligaments support the uterus. A hole in the middle allows menstrual blood to exit and sperm to enter. This passage is lined with secreting cells, which help to create the moist natural state of your vagina. And it is this very slim canal that dilates widely enough to deliver a baby.

Usually, the cervix is very firm. It subtly responds to hormones, growing more or less soft at opportune times. It's softest during ovulation, because that smart gatekeeper wants to let sperm through to meet the egg in the outer third of your tubes. The discharge of the endocervical glands changes throughout the cycle also. It's most supportive of sperm movement during ovulation, while after the event, the discharge is viscous and harder to swim through.

THE CELLS OF THE CERVIX
(IT'S MORE INTERESTING THAN IT SOUNDS)

Scientists and physicians have a good understanding of the complicated surface of the cervix. Most of the cervix is covered in squamous cells—comparable to the cells that cover your whole body—while the cervical canal is lined with columnar cells. These are very different. The squamous cells are fifteen to twenty cells thick, while the columnar cells are only one layer. Under a microscope, squamous cells look like a cobblestone street, while columnar cells look like a picket fence. Squamous cells are protective while columnar cells secrete mucus.

Where the squamous cells meet the columnar cells is called the S-C (squamo-columnar) junction. Every girl is born with a native

Nabothian Cysts

These occur on the cervix when a columnar cell, exposed on the outside of the cervix, is overrun by squamous cells. This lonely columnar cell continues to do its job-making secretions, which causes a small, painless bubble on the cervix that doctors call a Nabothian cyst. Almost all of them disappear, while the small remainder will hang out indefinitely and unobtrusively on the cervix. Just ignore them.

A virus is an organism that requires a host cell, unlike bacteria, which are totally self-contained and able to reproduce, excrete, breathe, metabolize, and grow. A virus has incomplete DNA and must latch onto other DNA to complete its essential functions – primarily reproduction. When the initial cell grows to a critical size, it explodes and thousands of new viruses have to look for host cells.

S-C junction right at the beginning of the cervical canal. This border remains visible for our entire lives, but with puberty, pregnancy, and sometimes systemic contraception, the cervix swells in response to different or increased hormones. This pushes the native S-C junction out to where a physician can readily see it, exposing columnar cells to the vagina.

Columnar cells are not happy in the vagina. There's lots of stuff they're not used to: the PH is different, the bacteria are plentiful, and there can be all sorts of foreign objects coming at them, like penises and tampons. To protect themselves, they begin a process called squamous metaplasia (*meta* means change, *plasia* means cells). This is when all the exposed columnar cells literally transform or mutate into squamous cells. So squamous metaplasia is a normal, benign process in which the columnar cells exposed to the vagina by the maturing cervix transform themselves into squamous cells. This process continues on throughout our lives until menopause for one reason or another.

The area between a woman's native S-C junction (the one she was born with) and a relatively new S-C junction is called the "transformation zone." *This is where all cervical cancer begins.* Doctors speculate this is because columnar cells must regress to a more primordial cell type to transform into squamous cells. It's likely that the more primitive cell is very sensitive to viruses.

significant problems of the cervix

233

CERVICAL CANCER

The carcinogenic virus of the cervix is HPV—human papilloma virus. There are up to one hundred strains of known HPV, almost all of which are considered "low risk." These benign strains cause all kinds of warts—warts on your fingers, feet, or genitals. High-risk strains are those that are most likely to cause cervical cancer.

HPV is present in semen and on the surface of the genitals, and is transmitted via unprotected sex. It takes about three months from exposure for HPV to be detectable. With the exception of warts, it is an asymptomatic problem, but, in the right circumstances, can be very medically significant.

If the cervix happens to have recently expanded (due to puberty, hormone shifts, pregnancy, or many other reasons), columnar cells are exposed to the vagina while they transform themselves into squamous cells. In other words, there is active squamous metaplasia in the transformation zone. Should a man have the opportunity to ejaculate HPV-loaded semen right onto these fragile cells,

A Wrong Turn

The first scientific look at cervical cancer was done at the turn of the century in Denmark, where scientists began scrutinizing who was dying of cervical cancer. The highest incidence was among prostitutes and the lowest among married Jewish women. So these scientists asked, 'What's the difference between these Jewish women and those prostitutes?" Well, the Jewish women only had sex with circumsized men. So they blamed smegma! Smegma is the white cheesy stuff under the foreskin, among other places. This began the cross-religion trend of circumcisions worldwide. Unfortunately, these particular scientists remarkably overlooked the gross difference in number of sexual partners between prostitutes and married Jewish ladies (who were likely to be virgins marrying virgins), which we now know to be the real cause of the varying cancer rates. Since then, smegma has been vindicated.

@vaginas

that woman may be at risk for cervical cancer. The virus can attach to the early squamous cell and cause the DNA of that cell to mutate into something malignant.

The cervix is at the greatest risk during adolescence, which is why cervical cancer is typically a disease of young women. This is also why cervical cancer wasn't a tremendous women's health problem (except for prostitutes) until the modern era, not because women weren't having sex at a young age, but because they tended to be monogamous.

Today, about four thousand women get cervical cancer in the United States each year. Approximately four hundred thousand get it worldwide. Since HPV is so prevalent and asymptomatic, our best weapon against cervical cancer, and it's a good one, is the Pap smear. The American medical establishment has invested plenty of time, energy, and money into the Pap smear infrastructure, so much so that between 1940 and 1960, cervical cancer went from the number one gynecological cancer to third (behind ovarian and uterine).

A Pap smear obtains exfoliated cells off of the cervix with a small brush or spatula during a routine gynecological exam. The results of the smear are sent to a pathologist. She then extrapolates back to the cervix itself from the few cells on the slide. As wonderful as they are, Pap smears are just a screening test, not a diagnostic tool. In fact, a single Pap smear is only 60 percent accurate. Patients need to have three of them with at least one year in between to reach over 95 percent accuracy, which is why regular Pap smears are so important. Even then, Pap smears can tell you that there may be a problem, but not exactly what it is. Only a biopsy can say there is cancer for sure.

The gap between a mildly abnormal Pap smear and invasive cancer can be ten years or more. An annual Pap smear will almost always detect a problem at an early, treatable, fertility-preserving, health-maintaining stage of the disease. So get your annual Pap smear, especially after a new sexual partner.

Pap smears are graded in terms of "class," which carry different treatment protocols. Varying regions, hospitals, and doctors use different terminology:

significant problems of the cervix

235

Pap Smear Grade	Alternate Terminology		Which means what?
I	Normal Tissue		Negative
II	Cellular Atypia	ASCUS = Atypical Squamous Cells of Undetermined Significance	The cells do not look quite right. Most physicians would follow up with a virapap to determine the presence of HPV.
IIIA	Mild Dysplasia	CINI = cervical intraepithelial neoplasia	Low Grade SIL = Squamous Intraepithelial Lesion (i.e. SIL)	This when the top third of the new squamous epithelium on the cervix is abnormal.
IIIB	Moderate Dysplasia	CINII	High Grade SIL	The top two-thirds of the squamous epithelium on the cervix are abnormal.
IIIC	Severe Dysplasia	CINIII	High Grade SIL	The entire squamous epithilium is abnormal.
IV	Carcinoma in Situ	CINIII	High Grade SIL	Virtually the same as IIIC, i.e. almost cancer
V	Invasive Cancer		Cancer of the Cervix

If you have an abnormal Pap result, the next step varies depending on how abnormal it is. Most abnormal Paps call for a virapap, meaning a test for the presence of HPV. This may change as our understanding and the prevalence of HPV grow, but today, without HPV, a Class II Pap result is of less concern, and the doctor would probably advise a follow-up Pap in three months. With HPV and a Class II Pap result, most physicians would recommend a colposcopy (like a pair of binoculars that magnify the cervix) on the outside chance that the Pap missed something. Depending on which strain of HPV the patient has (high or low risk), her risk of cervical cancer can be more readily assessed. Any Class III or worse result should be colposcoped, regardless of HPV.

For most physicians, the colposcope is a tool to assist in the gathering of tissue for a biopsy. While some oncologists are skilled enough to visually diagnose cervical disease, most gynecologists use the colposcope to see the transformation zone (see page 232) and any possible lesions. The gynecologist gathers cells from these specific places by pinching a little tissue (with a tiny hole puncher) to send to the pathologist.

After the biopsy, the physician performs an endocervical curettage (ECC) which will reveal any abnormality inside the cervical canal that your doctor cannot see. This involves scraping the inside of the cervix with a tiny curette (a slim, flexible spoon). Unfortunately, this hurts for about ten seconds. This material is also sent separately to the pathologist, so he can specifically report on the cervical cells both in the canal and outside of it. This can determine how your doctor continues your treatment.

If you have atypia or mild dysplasia on your biopsy (meaning the cells outside the cervix), and your ECC is negative (meaning there is nothing abnormal inside the cervix), then your doctor might recommend simply watching the cervix. Ninety percent of atypia reverts to normal on its own. Seventy percent of mild dysplasia reverts to normal within a year. For these patients, "watching

We've done a terrific job combating cervical cancer in this country, but things are very different in developing nations. There are women in certain parts of the world who finally come to the hospital only when the smell of their rotting tumor is so bad their families kick them out. Without an excellent medical infrastructure, Pap smears are unheard of or extremely difficult to organize effectively. A woman comes into the closest city from a village, she gets a Pap, and three months later, the doctor can't find her to deliver the results. Now, physicians in developing countries are experimenting with a procedure in which they shine a flashlight on a women's cervix, splash a little vinegar on it and whatever turns white, they burn off with a cautery. The vinegar tends to turn dividing cells white (like hydrogen peroxide on a cut). Of course, this falls far short of Pap smears in terms of precision, but many of these doctors don't even have the electricity to do most of our standard procedures. In a very short time they have dramatically reduced the incidence of cervical cancer with this primitive, minor surgery.

the cervix" means repeating Pap smears every three months and reevaluating their status in a year. In any lesion more advanced than a Class IIIA Pap, the patient must be treated more aggressively.

TREATMENT OF CERVICAL PRECANCER

The most common procedure for treating cervical dysplasia is a LEEP (a loop excisional electrocautery procedure). A white-hot, u-shaped wire shaves the surface of the cervix, removing the whole transformation zone and providing a nice, flat tissue sample to send to the pathologist. This is quick and can be performed in a doctor's office with local anaesthetic, though some doctors and patients prefer sedation in an operating room setting. There's no bleeding, because as the physician collects the tissue, the remainder is cauterized. The cervix heals from the inside out, so abnormal cells are not buried.

The LEEP is the standard for cervical dysplasia, as long as the ECC (see page 237) is negative. There are a few experts with the LEEP who can confidently use this technique for treatment of severe dysplasia, even in the face of a positive ECC. Usually, though, if the ECC is positive, meaning that there are abnormal cells deep within the cervix, doctors perform a cone biopsy. In this procedure, the doctor makes a circular incision around the cervical opening and cones it in, meaning that the removed tissue is shaped like a cone. This is performed in the hospital under anesthesia, and almost all patients leave the same day. However, cone biopsies are particularly linked to increased risk of future cervical incompetence or stenosis (see page 240).

Cryotherapy used to be a popular method of treating precancerous cervixes, but it is no longer the favored technique. In this procedure, the cervix is frozen, destroying the transformation zone and killing dysplastic cells. As the cervix heals after this procedure, it falls in on itself, dangerously hiding any abnormal cells deep in the cervical canal. This makes diagnosing a recurrence or persistence very difficult.

Laser also enjoyed a period of brief popularity in treating dysplasia, where doctors would literally vaporize the transformation zone.

NEWSFLASH
....

About ten strains of HPV are considered high risk. Strain #16 accounts for 50 percent, and strain #18 causes an additional 25 percent of all incidences of cervical cancer. There are two new vaccines in the works currently; one prevents strain #16 alone, and the other works against both high risk strains. Vaccines only work before one has been exposed to the virus, so this shot would have to be administered to people before they were sexually active (i.e. if you're reading this, it's probably too late for you). There's almost sure to be a debate about at what age we give children a vaccine against a sexually transmitted disease.
....

Cervical cancer is a disease of young women. It is a very significant risk for adolescents who have immature cervixes and are sexually active—especially if they do not practice safe sex. The cervical cancer poster girl is Evita Peron, which jibes with the often repeated rumor that she was a prostitute at an early age. She died at the tender age of thirty-three.

The problem with this method is that there is no tissue to send to the pathologist, and therefore no proof that the patient is cured. It's also exorbitantly expensive and not any better than less expensive and probably more accurate procedures.

Should a patient miss the boat on all the other possible avenues of treatment due to a long vacation from thinking and end up with microinvasive cervical cancer, she will usually need a simple hysterectomy. But as long as you get annual Pap smears, you shouldn't have to worry.

THE INCOMPETENT AND OVERLY COMPETENT CERVIX

During pregnancy, the mighty cervix is responsible for holding the fetus inside the uterus. The elastic fibers and connective tissue are usually strong and stretchable enough for this task. A weak cervix (doctors call this "incompetent") dilates painlessly and prematurely in pregnancy, and when the weight of the fetus grows (at about twenty to twenty-eight weeks), it can begin to fall out of the uterus without contractions. On the other end of the spectrum is cervical stenosis, which is when the cervix is too strong and refuses to dilate in labor. Thankfully, both these conditions are very rare (about 0.5 percent of pregnancies encounter one of these problems).

With adequate prenatal care, neither of these conditions should cause any real problem in the pregnancy. An incompetent cervix is diagnosed in the early second trimester, and is generally treated with a big stitch in the cervix to help keep it closed. The most obvious predictor of an incompetent cervix is a previous, painless, early, vaginal delivery. Cervical stenosis is diagnosed when the cervix remains unchanged over a subjectively defined length of active labor, though doctors also tend to be concerned when the cervix remains unchanged in the weeks leading up to delivery. Once it is clear that the cervix will not dilate, the only choice is a cesarean section.

Cervical incompetence and stenosis are unpredictable before pregnancy, and there are few ways to avoid them. These cervical issues can be congenital problems, but any cervical manipulation or procedure, will statistically increase the risk of both. Multiple D&C's, abortions, or other cervical procedures (e.g. a LEEP or cone biopsy; see page 238) can incidentally weaken or scar the cervix. It seems that the more times you tamper with the cervix, the more likely it is that it will not function properly.

CERVICITIS

This is an infection of the cervix, most commonly caused by chlamydia or gonorrhea, but any infection of the vagina can involve the cervix. Cervicitis causes the cervix to look red, inflamed, and pussy, but there are few symptoms. Patients sometimes notice increased discharge, or, in bad cases, vague discomfort. This problem is taken care of when the primary issue (the vaginitis, for example) is cured.

* * * * *

DAUGHTER: "So the cervix is a muscle?"

MOTHER: "Nope."

DAUGHTER: "It's an organ?"

MOTHER: "Ummm, sort of."

DAUGHTER: "Well what is it, exactly?"

MOTHER: "It's a cervix."

DAUGHTER: "So, it's just a cervix. That's it. Nothing else like it in the body."

MOTHER: "Pretty much."

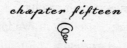

chapter fifteen

SIGNIFICANT PROBLEMS
OF THE VAGINA
AND EXTERNAL GENITALIA

Late one night I found myself watching the HBO show Real Sex, which I frankly find fascinating. This particular episode was about fake genitalia models; i.e. a man whose penis is used to make dildos and a woman whose vagina is reproduced in plastic (is there a name for such a thing?). The extremely professional male model had to maintain his erection for three minutes while cold plaster was poured into the cast around his dick. Meanwhile, a "fluffer" got the female model all excited and flushed before slapping some cold plaster on her external genitalia.

After all this hard work, the woman reaped the financial benefits at a local "gentlemen's club." She followed her feature performance with a crotch signing. Patrons stood on line, as at a book store, for her to sign a flesh-colored cheek. You might wonder, as I did, "What makes her vagina so special?" It is hairless, a nice rosy color, and symmetrical, but, most importantly, this vagina is available twenty-four hours a day, seven days a week to anyone with thirty bucks.

A fortune in time and money is spent agonizing over vaginal discharge, making it arguably the most significant problem of the vagina. True, unusual discharge can be a symptom of a problem or glitch in the natural homeostasis of the vaginal environment, but more often than not, women needlessly obsess over their vaginas and the healthy discharge therein. Gynecologists are constantly drawn into detailed discussions about the smell, volume, consistency, color, and taste. "It's a whitish yellow green." "It's a greenish yellowy white." "It's foamy bubbly." "It smells like shit." "It smells fruity." "It smells like something died." "It smells like fish." The truth is if it doesn't itch, burn or smell REALLY bad, discharge is almost definitely not problematic.

Sometimes, vaginas can go from smelling fine to smelling terrible, and this can be a sign of infection. *Vaginitis* is the catchall phrase for vaginal infection (*-itis* means infection) and it's practically an epidemic. The four varieties of vaginitis are fungal, viral, bacterial, and chemical.

FUNGAL (YEAST) INFECTIONS

Yeast is a very general, lay term for myriad strains of fungus that fall under the yeast category. Medical terms for yeast, or as they say in Italy, *fungi*, include Candida and Monilia. All of the strains are virtually the same in terms of symptoms and treatment options, so there is little reason to diagnose or discuss each type in particular, unless the patient's case is particularly bad (e.g. there are strains that resist antifungal medications). Should there be any need to diagnose a fungal infection, a vaginal culture (where a swab of discharge is put in a petrie dish to see what grows) can reveal exactly what strain of yeast is growing too big for its britches.

But Then, You're Lucky to Own a Vagina

. . . .

The worst thing you can have vaginally is no vagina. Vaginal agenesis—no vagina—is a congenital, highly unusual problem. Some women have two vaginas (called a double vagina), and wonder why their tampons don't work. Both of these problems can only be corrected with plastic surgery. So if you're reading this and you have one fully functional vagina, you're lucky.

. . . .

Yeast is a fungus and funguses like warm, moist, dark places—sounds just like a vagina to me. If you were a fungus, you'd love to live in a vagina. No surprise then that 100 percent of women have yeast present in their vaginas. Yeast also tends to thrive in higher acidity (i.e. low PH) environments and high sugar environments. Bacteria are also present in a healthy vagina (like acidophilus or lacto bacillus) to naturally keep the yeast in check. So a yeast infection happens when a normal inhabitant manages to become prevalent enough to cause symptoms.

These can range from tingly discomfort to mind-blowing burning itchiness accompanied by a cheesy discharge. The most common, minor yeast infections are the little itch many women notice two or three days before their period. The PH in the vagina drops throughout the cycle, making it most hospitable for yeast just before menstruation. When the period comes, the itch goes away.

Should the yeast come to dominate all its natural enemies in the vagina, discomfort can worsen to the point where you want to get a knitting needle, stick it up your vagina, and scratch like hell. This situation can continue to worsen, from itch to burn and then into pain. A significant yeast vaginitis is accompanied by the most incredible curdy discharge, like milk left out on the counter for a month.

WHAT ARE THE CAUSES OF A YEAST INFECTION?

1. *Absence of competition.* Yeast lives in a nice steady state in the vagina, but when its natural enemy gets killed off, the fungus can grow wild. Antibiotics, which are meant to kill bacteria, can kill all the yeast fighters in your body along with all the bad bacteria that makes you sick. For example, if you take Cipro for diarrhea, you might end up with a yeast infection. So if you are prone to yeast infections, and are going to take antibiotics, you should proactively treat the yeast infection (see page 246).

2. *Heat.* Anything that heats up the vaginal walls will also promote more rapid fungal growth. Friction caused, for example, by sexual

intercourse will warm the walls of the vagina (think an Indian Burn). Occlusive clothing and synthetic fibers don't allow the vagina to breathe, which is why loose cotton panties are a good idea. This may not be fashionable right now (and maybe it never was) but if you get lots of yeast infections, consider ditching your tight, lacy, polyester number for a good old pair of Hanes.

3. *Moisture*. Yeast likes it moist and humid. So there's nothing like a good pair of sweaty tights to get that yeast growing. That's why it's called jock itch.

4. *Sugar*. Yeast thrives on a high blood sugar—it's their food of choice. Therefore, eating lots of sweets can promote a yeast infection. More sensitive women will find that carbohydrates (like beer) can bring also bring on a bout of uncomfortable yeast.

5. *Hormones*. The pill or pregnancy can contribute to yeast infections by increasing the acidity of the vagina.

DIABETES AND YEAST INFECTIONS
Gynecologists diagnose diabetes 50 percent of the time. When faced with a persistent yeast infection, a blood sugar test is always a good idea. Once diagnosed, female diabetics often know that a yeast infection is the first sign that their blood sugar is probably not where it should be.

TREATING YOUR YEAST INFECTION
The traditional treatment for a yeast infection is an antifungal topical preparation. There are many over-the-counter varieties including Monistat and Gynelotrimin, which involve tamponlike applicators and anywhere from a one- to seven-day treatment cycle. The cure rate for these courses is directly related to how many days you opt to use the medicine—i.e. the seven-day option provides the highest chance of curing the yeast infection, if it is applied all seven days. These treatments are in no way dangerous or problematic.

··

It is possible to catch a yeast infection, though it's highly unlikely. I had a patient whose husband had athlete's foot. Sure enough, every time she took a bath, she got a yeast infection. If your boyfriend is diabetic, or if he's chubby, he can get yeast in all the nooks and crannies around his penis, scrotum, and groin. With diabetics, the yeast thrives off of the high blood sugar on their skin, and with heavier gents, the warm, moist crevices are like a home away from home. Jock itch can also be transferred from crotch to crotch. All these guys should speak to their doctors about getting it treated, although some nice gynecologists will give their best patients prescriptions for two.

··

But these medications do cost money and some studies suggest that anywhere from 30 to 50 percent of women who buy them do not have yeast infections. The quiet obsession that many women share about their vaginal discharges often leads them to the pharmacy looking for a "solution." It's always a good idea, if you're inexperienced with yeast infections or if you're not sure you have one, to go to your doctor and have your vagina cultured.

The newest treatment for yeast is a prescription drug called Diflucan. The entire treatment cycle is supposed to be one pill, though most women end up taking a second pill a few days later. Diflucan is a great option for patients with persistent yeast infections, as they can take one pill every week to hold the yeast at bay. The pill is easier (no messy cream), but it is less immediate as the medication takes a day or two to get into the bloodstream and down to the vagina. Unlike the topical preparations, there's nothing soothing about it.

significant problems of the vagina and external genitalia

247

VIRAL INFECTIONS

HPV (ALSO PAGE 114) AND VENEREAL WARTS

The Human Papiloma Virus (HPV) is the most common sexually transmitted disease and, not surprisingly, the most common vaginal virus. The latest gynecological research suggests that an overwhelming majority of sexually active young women have this virus at some point and that it typically goes away on its own within a few years. There are over a hundred strains of HPV, some of which are considered high risk because they have been linked to cervical cancer (page 234). The rest are not of much medical concern.

Although we call them *low risk* because they are not fatal, there are strains of HPV that cause condylomata or venereal warts. These are characteristically cauliflower like in appearance, with a bulbously uneven texture. They can grow at the vaginal opening, on the labia, around the rectum, or anywhere at all in the perigenital area, and when they do appear, they can grow indefinitely.

Needless to say, the sooner one deals with warts, the better. Gynecologists use acid, lasers, or a cautery to burn them off. This is

To Tell or Not to Tell?

When a woman has venereal warts, and a new sexual partner, she morally has little choice but to tell the new guy or gal. She knows she could give him or her genital warts as well. But when patients have asymptomatic HPV, and demand to be tested, they then have to question whether or not they need to tell their partners. Figure that a recent study in Costa Rica followed college-age women for one year, within which time 50 percent developed HPV. Almost all of these women will never have a HPV-related problem. The current CDC (Center for Disease Control) guidelines are not to test for HPV unless there is an abnormal Pap smear, and this is what I recommend. If you do have HPV, it's not causing you harm and to know won't do anyone any good. And once you know what's in your vagina, there's a moral code—you have to tell.

Before AIDS, there was herpes, the major medical event of the eighties. It's bittersweet to reflect on what a big deal we made out of a disease that's generally not fatal. A patient once said to me, "Tell me it's cancer. Don't tell me it's herpes." Within the medical profession, herpes was significant because it proved conclusively that we had yet to conquer infectious disease. For the single folks, herpes put a lid on the sexual revolution.

done in the doctor's office and hurts for a few seconds. If that sounds unappealing, there are new topical treatments (one brandname is Aldara) that spur the immune system to take the warts on, but it takes much longer and with less definite results.

HERPES (ALSO PAGE 109)

The second-most-common vaginal virus is herpes. The primary and most infamous symptom of herpes is painful sores on the vagina, the external vaginal wall, the labia, etc. The first outbreak is the worst, as per usual with viruses. Exposure causes a general sick, achey, rundown feeling as the virus courses through the bloodstream. Meanwhile, you may find one tiny cold sore on your external genitalia, or the entire vaginal area can be covered with them.

Herpes hurts, it's miserable, and it's disgusting. But there are only three groups of people whose lives are threatened by the virus, all of whom share compromised immunity: 1) people on immuno-supressive therapy because of an organ transplant or chemotherapy; 2) people with AIDS; and 3) newborn babies.

If you are in good health and do not fall into any of the above groups, herpes is not the end of the world. It's really just a cold sore in another place. The stigma is the worst thing about it. People are afraid to say they have it, and that contributes to the feeling that you're the only one who does. But, trust us, many, many people have it.

significant problems of the vagina and external genitalia

249

Herpes and HPV are very contagious viruses. If you have an open lesion, you should not not **NOT** engage in sexual activity. If you do not have a lesion, your infection rate drops precipitously. And if you use a condom all the time, it's highly unlikely you'll give it someone else, but it's never 100 percent safe—here are people who "shed the virus" when they don't have outbreaks (called asymptomatic shedding) and regardless, your partner may come down with it despite all your efforts. I've had married couples where one spouse has herpes, and they've been married twenty years without the other partner getting it. And I've had other cases where, within one month of initiating a sexual relationship and with all the care taken in the world, the partner gets an outbreak.

The simple basic truth is that the better your immunity, the less frequent your outbreaks. Some folks have one outbreak and that's it. They didn't get rid of the virus, they're just controlling it. This has to do with sleeping well, eating right, exercising regularly, reducing stress levels, and all of the other things your mother told you to do.

BACTERIAL VAGINAL INFECTIONS

BACTERIAL VAGINOSIS

Bacterial vaginosis is a condition associated with an imbalance in vaginal inhabitants, much like yeast infections, only in this case, the culprit is the bacteria Gardenerella. When it's present in the proper relative amount, Gardenerella causes no problems. But when the bacteria dominate the contents of the vagina, it alters the PH, the odor, and the quality of the secretions. On the plus side, if Gardenerella is the cause of your problems, you didn't catch it from anybody—it's a simple imbalance of the natural proportions of your vagina, and you don't have to make any nasty phone calls. However, even though bacterial vaginosis is not an STD, it is much more common in women who are sexually active.

Gardenerella itself is not a problem, but in altering the PH balance, it can make women vulnerable to other infections and in pregnancy may increase the risk of premature ruptured membranes and labor. So, for pregnant patients, doctors prescribe metronidazole, an antibiotic that comes in gel (brandname Metrogel) or pill form (brandname Flagyl).

BACTERIAL VAGINITIS

Any bacteria (e.g. Strep, Staph, Klebsiella) can get into the vagina, causing bacterial vaginitis. Unlike yeast, there are no natural enemies in the vagina to these bacteria, so they quickly rage out of control and are usually associated with a very bad yellowish puslike discharge. It is important to culture these symptoms and figure out precisely what kind of bacteria has taken over down there.

The most common bacteria in this area are:

1. *Beta hemolytic streptococcus*, also called group B streptococcus (or, shorter still, GBS). GBS is a benign guest in the vagina, meaning that in 10 percent of vaginas that permanently host this bacteria, there are no symptoms. Although GBS can be caught sexually (anything can be caught sexually, including the common cold) it can also be picked up in swimming pools, saunas, life, etc. Once there, it is virtually impossible to get rid of.

If You're Getting Really Lucky
....
Even the healthiest of vaginas are only designed to do so much. If you're lucky, you know that sensation of having had a little more vaginal intercourse than you should have. You're a little sore and uncomfortable the next day. This should hopefully bring a smile to your face and remind you of what caused it.
....

This may sound unappealing, and it is when a woman is first exposed or if the GBS acts up. For the first few months, she could have the same symptoms as any other vaginitis (yellowy, pusy discharge). Outside of the initial period and occasional flare-ups, there are generally no symptoms.

The problem with GBS is, once again, pregnancy. If a patient has GBS and delivers vaginally, there is a small chance the baby will catch it on the way through, and this can cause a catastrophic infection for the newborn. Current CDC guidelines recommend culturing all pregnant women for GBS and treating it with intravenous antibiotics in labor. This does not kill all the GBS, but rather reduces it dramatically. Once the baby is born, the patient comes off the antibiotics and the GBS asymptomatically returns.

2. *Staphylococcus aureus*. Out of all the bacterial vaginitises, this is the most dangerous. Unfortunately, staph can live anywhere on the outside of the body, and if there's a break in the skin (an abrasion, a little scratch, etc.) staph can enter the blood stream and cause toxic shock syndrome. Most people who have developed this infection are men and postmenopausal women, so tampons are not the only culprit. However, very absorbent tampons can irritate the walls of the vagina, so that if staph is present, you are at risk for TSS. You cannot get TSS from a tampon unless there is staph aureus present. If you are petrified of this syndrome, ask for a staph aureus culture and use your tampons in peace.

Aside from the big two, there are an infinite number of bacteria that a woman can have in her vagina. If someone gives you oral sex and they've got a strep throat, you get a strep vagina. If someone is manually caressing you, remember the all-important rule—go from front to back. If there is some stimulation at the rectal area, and you put that finger back in the vagina, you are introducing bacteria from the rectum that do not belong in the vagina. This can cause a vaginal infection that will be smelly and unpleasant. Fortunately, most all vaginal bacteria

vaginas

All healthcare professionals have their pick for the most stinky smell in medicine. In gynecology, we know that the forgotten tampon is the worst smell in the world. Ten plastic bags and a full spray can of deodorant later, and the room where you removed the tampon is still unusable. Should you forget your tampon, don't be alarmed when it stinks upon removal.

can be treated with local antibiotic cream or systemic antibiotics, which a gynecologist will be happy to prescribe.

CHEMICAL VAGINITIS

Some women's vaginas are very sensitive to soaps or chemicals. They can get in a bubble bath, use a new shower gel, or try a different laundry detergent and develop redness and irritation in their vaginas. Foreign-body vaginitis can result from anything in the vagina that doesn't belong there, depending on what the object is, how clean it is, and how sensitive the woman is. These intruders can cause an overgrowth of the natural bacteria and attract additional germs from the external genitalia, making for a really bad smell and a foul pusy discharge. The classic example of this is sandbox vaginitis, common among little girls. Depending on the cause, doctors will recommend a behavioral adjustment (throw away that new detergent), topical anti-inflammatories, or antibiotics.

VAGINAL CANCER

Vaginal cancer is generally a malignancy of older women, with an average age at diagnosis of sixty. Only 1 percent of all genital cancers are vaginal. Usually its symptoms include vaginal bleeding or an abnormal Pap smear. Doctors treat this disease with radiation, surgery,

D.E.S. (diethelstilbestrol) is a synthetic estrogen that was administered in the mid 1940s to women with high-risk pregnancies to prevent miscarriage. When the daughters of these women entered their twenties, they faced a much higher than average risk of vaginal cancer, with a median age at diagnosis of nineteen. Don't worry, DES has long been pulled off the shelves.

or both. If caught in the early stages, vaginal cancer can be cured up to 90 percent of the time.

EXTERNAL GENITALIA

GRAVITY STRIKES

Our pelvic floor developed perfectly for a quadraped. Unfortunately, we gave that up millennia ago, and now the vagina, rectum, and bladder are all pulled upon by gravity every day of our bipedal lives. As the years go by, and as we run, cough, laugh, sneeze, and have babies, we are weakening our pelvic floor. The vagina is essentially a big hole that can ultimately drag everything that's attached (the bladder, uterus, and rectum) with it as it falls, which, to some degree, it almost inevitably will. This results in a bulge protruding from the vagina that can be as small as a cherry or as big as a plum. Diagnoses range from a small dropped bladder to a total uterine prolapse, which is when the entire vagina inverts and hangs between the legs with the uterus inside the dangling pouch.

The best treatment for all of these issues is to never have them in the first place. *Kegel religiously.* Strengthen those muscles to keep everything down there where it belongs. Also, be aware that high impact activity weakens the pelvic floor. Any exercise where both feet leave the ground (jumping jacks, running, etc.) will magnify the weight of your body when it reconnects with earth—this puts a huge amount of weight on the pelvic floor. Vaginal childbirth further traumatizes the vagina and its environs, which makes kegels even more important. Other contributing factors include obesity, recurring pulmonary problems that cause long bouts of coughing and sneezing, and chronic constipation, all of which increase the pressure on that pelvic floor.

If you live long enough, all women develop some form of incontinence—urinary and/or fecal. This is all because of weakening muscles and that bitch, gravity. Take solace in the fact that your sisters suffer also.

But there's hope. A whole new area of medicine called urogynecology specifically addresses the problems of prolapse and incontinence with innovative surgical techniques. These are safer, less invasive, and more effective than traditional surgical approaches.

For the elderly, the traditional treatment for prolapse is a pessary. This is much like a diaphragm. They're usually made of rubber or

False Vaginismus Alert

When I was a resident, we got a house call request. The male caller said he was stuck in his wife and couldn't get out. There was a hot debate among the residents—we didn't know if it was priapasm (the inability to relax an erection) or vaginismus (an intense muscle spasm of the vagina, which can hold a penis captive). These conditions are so rare, both the urology and gynecology residents were excited to see it first-hand. As hospital rules barred house calls, we had to insist they come to the emergency room. There were only about 3,000 hospital staff waiting to greet this unfortunate couple. The stretcher had one man at the head and four feet at the bottom. It turned out the woman had an old metal IUD shaped in an M, and one end was poking out of the cervix. The instrument hooked her husband's foreskin, preventing his exit. Ultimately, the urology resident reached all the way up into the vagina and snipped a little bit of foreskin, releasing the husband. They then removed the IUD and everyone went home.

It's good to be aware that whatever can happen to skin can happen to the external genitalia. Because an ingrown hair or pimple is on your labia, it's just the same as all other topical anomalies. You can treat an ingrown hair anyway you like–some may pick while others will leave it alone. Sebaceous cysts are big zits and are generally painless. The surface can be whiter than the underlying skin and sometimes they get infected, come to a head, and pop. Again, some will pick, others will not. More inconveniently, excema and psoriasis (clinically dry, itchy skin) are possible on the labia. A gynecologist or dermatologist can prescribe a cream for these issues.

latex; some look like doughnuts, others look like cubes or triangles. They wedge between the sacrum and the pubic bone, holding everything in. A gynecologist fits the patient for one, and some need to be professionally changed each month by a physician. Others can be taken out at night like dentures.

CANCER

It is possible to get cancer of the rectum, labia, or vulva, though this is an older woman's problem. Generally physicians are able to catch these at a precancerous stage, improving survival rates. Abnormal growths on the external genitalia (that are not warts or herpes) are the only symptom of these diseases. Treatment includes radiation, surgery, or both.

Gynecologists are only just learning that there may be a connection between HPV and all three of these cancers, but this research is in its infancy. It seems, though, that should you have any significantly abnormal Pap smear results that lead to treatment (a LEEP or worse, see page 238), it's a good idea to keep an eye on all the squamous cells (i.e. skin) of the genitalia.

@vaginas

Most people associate melanoma with the sun, so skin cancer of the genitalia seems counterintuitive. It is very unusual to have a melanoma on the vulva or rectum, but it's possible. Generally, women who have had melanomas on other parts of their bodies (that see more sun) have been advised by their dermatologists to clue in the gynecologist, so she can be on the look out for any suspicious growths down below. Should a doctor see an unusual skin lesion, she will take a sample and send it to a pathologist. Gynecologists treat melanomas of the external genitalia by referring the patient to a specialist in that area.

* * * * *

MOTHER: "Rumor has it that Cleopatra used camel dung as a contraceptive."

DAUGHTER: "You mean, she put camel crap in her crotch and that kept the men away."

MOTHER: "No. They would have sex with her with the camel crap."

DAUGHTER: "What kind if infections would that cause?"

MOTHER: "I don't know. It was so smelly, she killed herself with a snake."

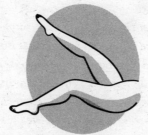

INDEX

myometrium, 3, 209
myths, common, 179–88

N
Nabothian cysts, 232
natural family planning, 93–94, 103
night sweats, 168
Nonoxynol 9, 85, 88
Norplant, 79, 101
nudity, xiv–xv
nutrition, during pregnancy, 154

O
oligomenorrhea, 21–24
oral contraceptives. *See* birth control pill
oral sex, 55–56
orgasms, xv, 57–62
    importance of, 61–62
    lack of, 57–58
    through masturbation, 58–60
    time for, 61
    vaginal, 60, 182–83
Ortho Tri-Cyclen, 84
osteoporosis, 32, 168–70
ovarian pain, 2, 185
ovarian problems, 191–206
    abscesses, 204–5
    functional cysts, 192–99
    miscellaneous, 204–6
    ovarian cancer, 201–4
    polycystic ovaries, 196–97
    tumors, 197–201
ovarian sparing, 205
ovaries
    about, 1–2
    birth control pill and, 37–38
    polycystic, 23
    radiation and, 38
    removal of, 219
ovulation
    about, 13
    during adolescence, 15–16
    conception and, 141–42

P
panties, 42
panty liners, 42
Pap smears, 34, 235–37
parasitic fibroids, 212
patch, 77, 99
pedunculated fibroids, 211
pelvic floor, weakened, 254–56
pelvic infections
    birth control pill and, 74
    Dalkon Shield and, 92
pelvic inflammatory disease (PID), 91, 107
penis size, 67
perimenopause, 166–67
perineal orifices, 4–5
perineum, 9, 47
period. *See* menstruation
peritoneum (serosa), 3
pessary, 255–56
PH levels, 24
pill. *See* birth control pill
pituitary gland, 12, 13, 71
Plan B, 80
platelets, 147–48
PMS (premenstrual syndrome), 18–21
polycystic ovaries, 23, 196–97
polyps, 227
post-pill suppression, 73
pre-eclampsia, 158–59
pregnancy
    See also miscarriages
    age and, 144–46
    alcohol use during, 150
    basics of attaining, 141–42
    bed rest during, 153
    birth control pill and, 83
    bleeding during, 152
    caffeine during, 150
    complications during, 158–59
    concerns during, 148–53
    detecting early, 146–47
    ectopic, 128, 148, 206–8
    fibroids and, 214–15

sexual positions, 55
sexually transmitted diseases (STDs)
    about, 105–6
    AIDS, 105, 116–20
    bacterial, 106–9
    birth control pill and, 75
    chlamydia, 106–7
    condoms and, 84–85
    gonorrhea, 106–7, 204–5
    hepatitis B, 115–16
    herpes, 109–14, 249–50
    HIV, 116–20
    human papilloma virus (HPV),
        74–75, 114–15, 180, 231,
        234–35, 239, 248–49
    lice, 122
    parasitic, 121–22
    preventing, 51–52
    syphilis, 107–9
    trichomonas, 121
    viral, 109–20
Sims, J. Marion, 59
smell, 41
smoking, 149
sonograms, 156–57, 192, 193
speculums, 33–34
spermicide, 85, 88, 103
spirochetes, 107
squamo columnar junction (S-C junc-
    tion), 4, 232–33
squamous epithelium, 4
squamous metaplasia, 233
staphyloccus aureus, 252
stirrups, 33
stroma, 2
submucous fibroids, 211
subserosal fibroids, 210–11
suction curettage, 126–30
surgical abortions, 126–30, 132
syphilis, 107–9, 110
systemic hormonal treatments, 70–84
    birth control pill, 71–77, 81–84
    effectiveness of, 99–100
    Lunelle, 78

morning after pill, 79–80
patch, 77, 99
progesterone pills, 78–79
progesterone shots, 79
ring, 78, 99

T
Tamoxifin, 226
tampons
    for teens, 27
    toxic shock syndrome and, 25–26
    for vaginal secretions, 42
    vs. pads, 26
Tay-Sachs, 142
teenagers
    on the pill, 82–83
    sex and, 62–65
tenaculum, 126
testosterone, 15, 201
toxemia, 158–59
toxic shock syndrome (TSS), 25–26
toxoplasmosis, 143
trichomonas, 121
tubal ligation, 95–98, 103
tumors
    fibroid, 210–16
    ovarian, 197–201
Tuskegee Study, 110

U
ultrasounds, 156–57, 192, 193
urethra, 5, 40
urine samples, 31
uterine ablation, 14
uterine cancer, 23
uterine prolapse, 254–56
uterine scarring, 129
uterus
    about, 3, 38, 209
    endometriosis and, 221–25
    fibroids in, 210–16
    hysterectomies and, 216–20
    sarcoma of, 220–21
    tipped, 223

vaginas

ABOUT THE AUTHORS

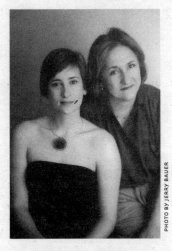

CAROL LIVOTI was born and raised in Brooklyn, New York. After attending college at Cornell University, she moved to Manhattan, which has been home ever since. She currently is in private practice in OB-GYN at Lennox Hill Hospital in New York. After her beautiful family and her career, her third love is traveling. She's married to Richard Topp and they have one child, Elizabeth.

ELIZABETH TOPP was born and raised in Manhattan. After attending Harvard College, Liz went on jaunts through Europe, Asia, Africa, Australia, and Austin, Texas only to end up back in New York City in the same apartment she grew up in. Liz has been Al Franken's assistant and currently works for Caroline Kennedy.